RETURN
TO
HEALTH

Overcoming the Unimaginable
and Beating the Odds

Dr. Robert Kuhn

BALBOA.
PRESS

A DIVISION OF HAY HOUSE

ISBN: 978-1-4525-5672-7 (sc)
ISBN: 978-1-4525-5673-4 (e)
ISBN: 978-1-4525-5674-1 (hc)

Library of Congress Control Number: 2012914472

Balboa Press books may be ordered through booksellers or by contacting:

Balboa Press
A Division of Hay House
1663 Liberty Drive
Bloomington, IN 47403
www.balboapress.com
1-(877) 407-4847

Because of the dynamic nature of the Internet, any web addresses or links contained in this book may have changed since publication and may no longer be valid. The views expressed in this work are solely those of the author and do not necessarily reflect the views of the publisher, and the publisher hereby disclaims any responsibility for them.

The author of this book does not dispense medical advice or prescribe the use of any technique as a form of treatment for physical, emotional, or medical problems without the advice of a physician, either directly or indirectly. The intent of the author is only to offer information of a general nature to help you in your quest for emotional and spiritual well-being. In the event you use any of the information in this book for yourself, which is your constitutional right, the author and the publisher assume no responsibility for your actions.

Any people depicted in stock imagery provided by Thinkstock are models, and such images are being used for illustrative purposes only.
Certain stock imagery © Thinkstock.

Printed in the United States of America

Balboa Press rev. date:09/24/2012

Contents

This book is dedicated to all the sick and suffering in the world. Never lose hope and never give up. As long as you have a breath in you, there is room for a miracle.

Foreword

There are thousands of really great physicians and health care providers in the world. I know, because I've met and talked with many of them in my twenty-plus years working in the field. As publisher of the *Chiropractic Journal*, head of Chiropractic Benefits Services, and author of wellness books like *Chiropractic Works!* and *Unleashed*, I've been blessed with the opportunity to make contact with some of the most successful and inspiring practitioners around today.

Within that vast crowd of exceptional men and women, a few stand out as true models for us all. These are the individuals who've both excelled in their field and have a gift for transforming the lives of those around them.

One member of that elite corps of extraordinary people is Dr. Robert Kuhn. I've known Rob for years, and I can't think of anyone more qualified to write a book on how to regain or optimize health. He's been there, done that. He managed to pull himself and his whole family back from the brink of disaster when they all faced a potentially fatal health condition. Ever since, he's dedicated his life to teaching others how they can do it too.

In this book he says, "I have never ever wanted to live an ordinary life. I want all the passion, pizzazz, power, and playfulness that life has to offer." That's Rob all over! The energy and commitment he demonstrates every day of his life makes him more than just an inspiration. He's living proof that we don't have to accept a verdict of illness or death imposed on us by the medical establishment. We can all take actions *now* to reverse the pattern of sickness and aging and live life with the passion, pizzazz, power, and playfulness that Rob enjoys.

Despite the dramatic story about his family's health problems, he never wallows in a pool of self-pity over past ills. He's risen above that narrative to write himself a new one that's full of health and happiness. It's the kind of story he wants his readers to be able to claim for themselves, and he tells them to "live your life with the intention of always having and creating good health." This book offers very specific and practical steps to help you do just that.

First, you need to overcome the brainwashing we've been subjected to about how great the traditional medical approach is—how drugs and surgery will cure anything. They won't, and Rob knows this firsthand. In this book—as in everything he does—he's totally honest and plainspoken about the good, the bad, and the downright ugly aspects of modern medicine. Never sugarcoating facts just so they'll go down easier, he gives it to you straight. That, too, is Rob all over!

The bottom line? The power to regain or optimize true health is in your own hands. Drugs and surgery won't make you well. Even Rob's book can't "cure" what's ailing you. Like the greatest healers of all time, he's a teacher rather than a medicine man. He shows you how to change your mindset, your diet, your lifestyle—and your "story." The result can be an incredible new pain-free lease on life that leaves you fit, strong, and healthy.

Rob often says it's his God-given mission in life to help people. With this book, he's definitely fulfilling that mission.

— Timothy Feuling

Introduction

You Can Regain
Your Health ... Really!

One thing I notice about the patients that come to see me in my practice is that whether they realize it or not, they are all looking for something more than pain relief. For the great majority of them, that something is a return to health. Bringing a sense that their bodies are breaking down and poor health is rapidly engulfing them, they want to recapture the vitality, vigor, and good health that seem to have long since left them.

Their bodies ache; they move slower; they feel uninspired about life; and they are taking numerous medications just to make it through each day. In most cases, just sitting in the exam room with them I can sense the weight of the world on their shoulders. Once minor, occasional health concerns have now turned into daily worries. Little aches and pains that used to appear only after overexertion or extra-long days at work now rear their ugly heads with great frequency. Obesity and immobility are the rule, not the exception.

Most people that I work with now are dealing with severe fatigue, some level of depression related to their poor health, and a smattering of health problems that range from acid reflux to migraine headaches. The number of people coming to my clinic who are taking high blood pressure medication and high cholesterol medication has skyrocketed over the last several years, and the number of people who have heart disease, cancer, or diabetes is absolutely mind-boggling. They are stressed out, burned out, and feel like they are just trudging along. For many of them, their sense of desperation could be cut with a knife.

Chronic conditions, such as Type 2 Diabetes, fibromyalgia, carpal tunnel syndrome, hypothyroidism, sciatica, headaches, irritable bowel and restless leg syndrome, are now affecting a large portion of the population. Autoimmune conditions are running rampant. Sadly, many of these patients have been misdiagnosed and mistreated. While such patients used to be few and far between, they are now commonplace.

Here's the kicker: the majority of people I am referring to here are under the age of fifty! What??? Yes, that's right. People under the age of fifty are in such poor health these days that it's almost inexplicable. How can this be? Doesn't the United States spend more money on healthcare and research than any country in the world? You bet we do! So how can Americans have such disgustingly poor health?

Believe it or not, the answer to that question is pretty simple, and understanding it can help you get your life back. While simple, it's not just as easy as saying, "Well, you just need to eat better food," although that's a great place to start.

My inspiration for writing this book is *you*! I assure you that contained in the pages of this book are the answers to why people in America are dying of sickness and disease faster than in any other industrialized nation in the world. But let's be honest—you, the reader, want to know what this book will do for you. My hope for you is that no matter what you are dealing with or where your current level of health is, reading this book will not only help you regain your health, but it will transform and inspire you and set you on the road to fulfilling a brighter future.

That might sound like a tall order to fill. After all, I don't know you and I don't know what particular problem you have. Maybe you just want to get a little healthier; maybe you want to lose weight; or maybe you are the worst of the worst. No matter where you rank on that list, I've seen it. The techniques and principles in this book have been instrumental in helping others just like you dramatically improve their lives.

In order for you to live at your highest optimal health potential, you not only must understand what you need to do, but you also need to understand which behaviors got you to where you are now. There is an unbelievable amount of misinformation and poor health advice out there right now. I am often blown away by some of the things my patients are trying to do to improve their health according to what they've Googled or what a friend or family member told them to do. You need the best information out there. You need the real thing! You need information that is based on proven research, the stuff with the power to change your life. While I don't claim to be able to heal every person on the planet (darn), I can definitely provide you with the info you need to make powerful, sweeping changes in your life and health.

To get started, it will be of tremendous benefit to you to know something about who I am and why I am the right guy to write this book. I myself was on what I truly felt was death's door, and I totally got my life back. In chapter 1, I will tell you about this in detail, and I won't hold back. I am going to tell you how my life was nearly destroyed through misdiagnosis and lack of knowledge. The remainder of this book will explain how I got my life back by practicing the same principles and techniques that I have been teaching my patients for over a decade. Whether you need inspiration, minor adjustments to your health, or a complete overhaul of your life, this book is for you.

I want you to know from the outset that I will not sugarcoat anything in this book. In fact, you may hear some things in this book that challenge everything you've ever known. Some points may be totally offensive to you. After all, sometimes the truth hurts. It doesn't happen very often, but on occasion I have had one or two attendees at my seminars get red-in-the-face mad at some of the assertions I have made against the medical industry. I can assure you the reason they were so upset is that my points were based on facts that nobody likes to hear.

Before we begin, I just want you to know that I respect your time, and I will do my best not to waste it. I have seen patients from all walks of life, dealing with the worst possible health scenarios, who completely got their lives back, and so can you. I believe in you. I believe in the healing power of your body, and I believe in miracles. If you truly want to change your health and reclaim your life, I believe that you can!! Let's get started.

PART I

Learning About Sickness

Chapter 1

Back from the Brink

There is one thing stronger than all the armies in the world, and that is an idea whose time has come.

—Victor Hugo

May 1, 2008

Today is my thirty-ninth birthday. It's 7:15 am, and I'm standing in the upstairs guest bathroom in my house. I'm staring at myself in the mirror. My skin is jaundiced, with a horrifying yellowish tint. My eyes are bloodshot, and I mean to the point where it looks like I stayed out until three o'clock in the morning drinking tequila. My arms tremble uncontrollably. In fact, my entire body is shaking mildly, and once again I feel nauseous. Every time I take a breath, it feels as though my lungs are filled with shards of crushed glass. I am cold and shivering, even though it's springtime. A splitting headache pounds my skull, and even though I just slept through the night, I feel like I need to be in bed for about another two days to regain some energy. My eyes begin to tear up as I look at myself and think, "Today is going to be the last day that I am alive on this planet."

It's time to go to work. Do I go to work or to the emergency room? This is a disturbing question to ask early in the morning. After three years of bouncing around from doctor to doctor trying to figure out why I was in this position and what was wrong with me, I knew that there was nothing medicine could do to help me. A whole lot of ghastly statistics and part of my life's work had told me that hospitals are places where sick people go to die. As bad as I felt, I chose to go to work. This is my story.

The Story Is Part of the Problem

In my first draft of this chapter, I wrote my story in its complete and total entirety. I included every painful detail. Feeling strongly about what my family and I went through, I wanted the world to know what happened point by point so that I could hopefully prevent others from suffering the same fate.

But by doing that I would be reinforcing one of the most negative, health-draining behaviors that people partake in: telling their stories. You see, everyone has a story. Everyone! And for most people, that story becomes a self-limiting crutch that prevents them from ever living a life of happiness.

"I'm depressed because my wife left me." "I'm not doing well at work because I'm not smart enough." "I can't make a relationship last because of my upbringing." The list goes on and on. While some of these things may be true, they are still a story, and they still hold you back. For many people there is a huge payoff in holding on to those stories. Sometimes they receive attention from others for telling their sad story. Other times their story allows them to be taken off the hook, to not face the truth about why something isn't working in their life. It doesn't matter what kind of payoff it is. A payoff is a payoff, and it could seriously hinder your chances of regaining your health or achieving your dreams.

Let me give you some examples of people's stories that relate to their health. These are things I hear on a daily basis; they keep people from actually being able to achieve the level of health that they want:

- I have fibromyalgia, so …

- I'm overweight because …

- My MS is causing …

- I can't do this because …

- I can't exercise because …

- My thyroid causes …

- I have peripheral neuropathy, so …

- My migraines cause me to …

- My back will never be better because …

- My parents had this so …

- This has been going on ever since …

This is just a short list of the stories I hear in my practice on a regular basis. To be clear, I'm not saying that people don't actually have these conditions, because they do. I'm also not saying that these conditions don't present challenges, because they do. The problem is that for many, the condition becomes their story, and once they have a story it can be a major obstacle to healing.

When I hear a sentence begin that way, I know someone is about to tell me their story again. Here's the issue: while it may be true that you have fibromyalgia, MS, or peripheral neuropathy, believing your own story inhibits you from moving forward in your life. Your story becomes your identity. You must change it!

Let me give you an example. I had a fifty-year-old female patient a few years back who had been diagnosed with fibromyalgia, which is a condition of global body pain. We'll call her Michelle. Michelle had completely bought into her diagnosis, hook, line, and sinker. She always came into the office with the statement, "My fibromyalgia is killing me today." One day she came in shaking and upset. She walked very slowly with a cane and made a scene over how much pain she was in. In a very loud, shaky, and upset tone, she said to me, "I'm having a terrible fibro flare-up." As a matter of fact, she told everyone else in the office too—the other patients, my staff, anyone who would listen. Here is the really interesting part of the story. She was my last patient on the morning shift that day. About fifteen minutes after she left, I went to a café right around the corner from my office to get some lunch. I walk into the café, and who did I see laughing, joking, and walking swiftly through the restaurant without a cane or any apparent physical disability? You guessed it. My patient Michelle appeared to be in no pain and to be having a great time. Of course, I would like to say it was because the treatment that she just received was so incredibly awesome, but there's more to it than that.

Am I suggesting that while in my office she was faking it? It's hard to say, but consider this. When she was in my office, her husband was with her. He coddled her and looked very concerned, obviously stressed over her condition. When I saw her at the restaurant, her husband wasn't there. She was there with a few other ladies having lunch. You can decide for yourself what the difference was.

Psychologically speaking, people get affirmation, a feeling of significance, and other types of emotional support from clinging to their story. They may not even realize that they are telling their story for those reasons, but that's why they do it.

Now, back to me. Because it became a major hindrance to my own healing, I have moved past my story. I don't particularly want to tell it anymore, but for you to understand where I'm coming from as well as my approach to helping you return to health, it is important for you to know my story. That said, I'm going to give you the Cliff's notes version so you can understand the challenges I faced and how I overcame them.

August 15, 2005

This was both a bittersweet and exciting day for us as a family. Tired of the rat race of big-city life and months on end of sweltering Phoenix heat, we were on our way to a new life in Virginia. My wife and I were leaving behind a beautiful home that we had moved into two years earlier, some great friends, my parents, and a six-year-old thriving practice that we had built from the ground up. With a huge vision of a new life in a smaller town, four seasons, green grass, and unlimited possibilities, we headed for Williamsburg, Virginia.

The move-in period was smooth, as usual. My wife and I are great planners (especially Wendy), and this was the third move we had made together as a couple, so we pretty much had it down pat. Staying true to form when we moved in, we had everything unpacked, pictures hung on walls, blinds hung up and the house completely ready and open for business in less than forty-eight hours after our arrival. This usually blows our new neighbors away, but, hey, that's how we roll.

In late November of 2005, just a few months after moving in, I noticed that I began to have some strange health symptoms. It started out innocently enough with minor bouts of dizziness, occasional headaches, and some shortness of breath. That "innocently enough" quickly snowballed into a health nightmare. Within a year, my list of ailments included:

- Daily chest pain

- Daily nausea

- Disturbances in body temperature (sometimes hot, sometimes cold)

- Stabbing abdominal pain

- Dry, scaly-looking skin

- Nosebleeds

- Daily sore throat

- Muscle pain

- Cramping

- Severe fatigue

- Memory loss

- Night sweats

- Swollen lymph nodes

- Depression

- Ringing in the ears (tinnitus)

- Powerful heart palpitations

- Weird skin rashes

- Muscle tremors

- Visual disturbances

- Constant redness of the eyes

- Tachycardia (racing heartbeat)

The worst part of it all was that it wasn't just me. My entire family was suffering from a combination of all of these problems. It is very disturbing to have your wife and kids sick without knowing why or how to fix it. Although my list of health problems continued to grow, I didn't go to a doctor for the first several months. Why? Because I had a sneaking suspicion that if I did go, they would run a plethora of tests and then come back and tell me everything was normal. Guess what happened when I did finally go to the doctor? Yep, you guessed it. A whole bunch of tests, and they didn't find anything. Predictably, when they couldn't find anything wrong, they offered me antidepressants and insinuated several times that it must all be in my head or related to stress. Thinking about it now still ticks me off. I know that this scenario sounds all too familiar to many of you, because you've experienced it yourself. *Fear not*! I'm going to show you why this happens.

The long and short of it was that within about eighteen months of moving to Virginia my wife and I and all three kids became terribly ill, and nobody could figure out why. In that time, we were misdiagnosed, not diagnosed, and were pretty much perceived as hypochondriacs with extreme anxiety.

Knowing that we weren't crazy, we continued to do our own research. Finally, after over two years of struggle, stress, and heartbreak, God gave us the big break we needed. We were watching a show called *Mystery Diagnosis* on television one night. We had never seen it before, so it had to be divine intervention that Wendy put it on. Not coincidentally, the episode featured a woman who was suffering from the exact same problems as us. As we watched, we were dumbfounded about how similar our stories were. Her diagnosis: toxic black mold poisoning. The rest, as they say, is history. The next day we called for a mold inspection of our beautiful brand new home, and, sure enough, toxic black mold was found in several areas of our house, including the entire crawl space, which meant it had gotten into the air conditioning as well. Day in and day out, we were constantly breathing a deadly biotoxin.

It was horrifying, but we had an answer. Now we could figure out how to get well. Unfortunately, one of the brilliant medical doctors I saw told me that if you are exposed to black mold, you die from it. How's that for taking away hope? Well, we knew better. Natural healthcare physicians have always worked under the premise that if you can find the cause of a health problem, then you can heal from it. My wife and I worked our butts off to get our family healthy again, and we succeeded.

During those three years of trying to figure out what was wrong with us, we were under the care of some of "the best" doctors, the most highly recommended, with the best credentials, who everyone raved about as being the best in town. Not one of them had a single clue about what was wrong with us! MRIs, CT scans, diagnostic ultrasounds, upper GIs, lower GIs, twenty different panels of blood work and *not one of them* ever even mentioned the possibility that we could be suffering from mold poisoning!

You ever notice that everyone thinks he or she has the best doctor? Think about it. When was the last time you were at a dinner party and you heard somebody exclaim, "Oh, my pediatrician is the absolute worst!" No. I see it in my practice every day. "Dr. Rob, I have to go get this procedure done, but I'm going to so-and-so; he's the best, you know." "Dr. Rob, I have to get this test done, but I'm going to so-and-so. She's the best in the state, you know." We all think we have the best doctor, yet day after day, year after year, we become sicker and sicker, taking more and more medications, all under the care of the best doctors. Hmmm, that's perplexing, don't you think?

The point of all this is that when it comes to chronic health problems, I truly know how you feel. I understand the frustration. I understand the hopelessness. I know what it's like to spend time and money, only to get zero results and I know the desperation of feeling like you don't have a future. I get it, and I'm here to show you how to get your life back.

Blazing a New Trail

In the world of healthcare, there is a new sheriff in town, and his name is *functional medicine*. Functional medicine saved my family's life, and it has helped me to change the lives of countless numbers of people over the years in my practice. Amazingly, the majority of people in our country still don't know what functional medicine is and have never even heard the term before.

Straight from the website of the Institute for Functional Medicine (www.functionalmedicine.org/), here's a textbook definition of what functional medicine is:

Functional medicine addresses the underlying causes of disease, using a systems-oriented approach and engaging both patient and practitioner in a therapeutic partnership. It is an evolution in the practice of medicine that better addresses the healthcare needs of the 21st century. By shifting the traditional disease-centered focus of medical practice to a more patient-centered approach, functional medicine addresses the whole person, not just an isolated set of symptoms. Functional medicine practitioners spend time with their patients, listening to their histories and looking at the interactions among genetic, environmental, and lifestyle factors that can influence long-term health and complex, chronic disease. In this way, functional medicine supports the unique expression of health and vitality for each individual.

In lay terms, this is saying that functional medicine serves to actually find and fix the root cause(s) of a patient's health problem, whereas traditional Western medicine only focuses on addressing symptoms.

Functional medicine utilizes a wide variety of testing, both medical and alternative, to locate the actual cause of a health problem. Those tests may include traditional blood tests as well as nontraditional tests, such as testing stool samples for parasites or bacterial infections, accurate food sensitivity testing, hair analysis, organic acid tests, hormone testing, adrenal stress index testing, and more.

The goal of most traditional medical care is to get a patient past an acute phase of symptoms, without real thought given to the future. The goal of functional medicine is to find out why the patient is having the symptoms, fix the problem, and set the patient up for a future of health and vitality. Which approach would you rather rely on?

I'll give you a prime example. If a patient having chest pains goes to a cardiologist and the doctor discovers that one of the coronary arteries is blocked, the doctor will most likely insert a stent into the artery. This procedure will alleviate the patient's chest pain and, in the short term, will be a very beneficial and even life-saving event. However, just inserting a stent doesn't address the problem of why the patient's artery became blocked in the first place. Most patients in this situation will be given a handout that tells them to stay away from saturated fats, and that's about it. Many of these patients will end up back at the doctor's office again, needing another stent and accumulating further coronary damage. I had a patient like this in Phoenix. He had a stent in every one of his coronary arteries by the time he was sixty years old. I haven't seen him in about eight years, and I sometimes wonder if he is still alive.

If the same patient showed up with chest pain in my office, I would refer him to a cardiologist for evaluation and the stent if necessary, instructing him to return to me afterward so we could fix his health problem and prevent any further coronary damage. I would subsequently do a whole body assessment to better understand why he developed a clogged artery to begin with. That might mean addressing his blood sugar levels, gut function, adrenal glands, thyroid gland, hormones, and, of course, lifestyle. I would have that patient complete a food diary for me so that I could gain a total understanding of how he had been living his life and teach him how to change it. I would recommend a specific exercise program for him and coach him on a weekly basis. My goal would be nothing short of teaching this man how to regain his health and reach a point of total vitality to live the life of his dreams. If that explanation sounds like what you are looking for, you're reading the right book at the right time!

When I began practicing chiropractic in 1999, I counseled patients on weight loss, nutrition, exercise, stress management, proper sleeping habits, empowering beliefs, nervous system health, and detoxification. At that point in time, even I had not heard the term *functional medicine*, but I was a functional medicine doctor without realizing it.

In the beginning, my methods were crude, to say the least. My recommendations for care were based on a thorough orthopedic and neurological evaluation, new patient questionnaires, and health history. Clinically speaking, there is nothing wrong with that, but when I consider the level of testing and methods I utilize today, I was in the crawling stage at best back then.

Over the years I have continued to learn and grow. My vision for how I practice healthcare has changed considerably. While I am extremely proud to be a doctor of chiropractic, my practice goes way beyond that. I am now a full-fledged functional medicine doctor with a Board Certification in Integrative Medicine. I now focus on taking care of chronically ill people. Some of my patients have tried everything else and failed. When it comes to being sick, the bottom line is that you want results. Am I right? That's the best part about functional medicine. The limited number of doctors out there who practice this way get results like no other. It is amazing to see what we can do for people who have been suffering from chronically poor health for years. The beautiful part of it is that everything I do is all natural and completely in line with my philosophy of healthcare.

Utilizing these methods that have stood the test of time, combined with newer strategies in functional medicine, helped my family regain our health. We have made a recovery that few mold patients ever see, and it is all due to following functional medicine protocols. (Note: Functional medicine is not the same as traditional medicine. I do not want to misrepresent myself. I am not a medical doctor.)

How Does This Affect You?

Because you have decided to invest your time and money in reading this book, I am assuming that you want more for your health. You have probably read other books or done research on the Internet. You may have even been to other alternative health care doctors, like chiropractors, acupuncturists, or a naturopath. Good for you! You have already done more than most people are willing to do to change their lives.

I have written this book in two parts: learning about sickness and returning to health. The truth is, you cannot create ultimate health in your body without first knowing what causes utter disaster in your body. Sadly, a big part of the problem in our country is following the "normal" healthcare path. (You will see what I mean in the next chapter.) In part two of the book, we will begin putting you back together in a new and healthy way. I will show you how to climb to levels of health that you never thought possible; if you'll follow my lead, your vitality will shine.

A huge part of what I do in my practice is to help people overcome chronic health conditions, autoimmune problems, and alarmingly poor health. I expect that many such people will be reading this book. If you are not someone suffering from a chronic health problem but are just interested in increasing your health and longevity, take this to heart: overcoming poor health and creating optimal health are one in the same. This book will be just as valuable to someone who is physically fit, eats right, and maintains good health, as it will be for someone with fibromyalgia or lupus.

My goal is that by reading this book you will not only gain a better understanding of what needs to be done to truly release the health that is within you, but that you will look back sometime in the future and realize that this book helped you make major changes in your life. I am and always have been a terrific dreamer. I have never ever wanted to live an ordinary life. I want all the passion, pizazz, power, and playfulness that life has to offer. Hopefully you are someone that wants to elevate your life to another level as well. What level is that? Only you can answer that question, but I hope it means that you want more: more health, more happiness, more time, and more fulfillment.

It should help to know that you are receiving a message from someone who has been there and done that. I know that what I do works for several reasons. One, for years I've seen the principles that I'm going to teach you produce life-changing results in my practice. Two, I belong to a group of the best functional medicine doctors in the world; I see these methods changing the lives of thousands of people in their practices as well. Three, these methods saved my family's life from toxic mold poisoning. Finally, I believe that it is my God-given mission in life to help you.

You'll notice that I include action steps to follow at the end of each chapter in part two. I'd ask that you implement at least one of the action steps from each chapter in your life—at least one. The more you implement, the better your health is going to get. Changing your life takes action. If you are willing to take massive action, you will reach new heights that you never thought possible. Let's begin.

Chapter 2

The Downfall

If you took all the medicine on the planet and threw it in the ocean, it would be good for humanity and bad for the fish.

—Dr. Charles Mayo (founder of the famed Mayo Clinic)

The Miracle of Medicine

Several years ago I saw a segment on a news television show about how a team of doctors separated a pair of Siamese twins who were joined together at the sacrum. The entire process was nothing short of absolutely amazing.

The sacrum is the center of your pelvis, which most people would refer to as the tailbone. If you know anything about anatomy, you know that the sacrum is dense with nervous system tissue. The majority of the lumbosacral plexus exits from the sacrum, which carries a wealth of nerves and blood supply. This is an incredibly delicate area of the body; if anything went wrong, disastrous outcomes, such as paralysis or death, could result.

I watched in awe as a team of doctors performed this miraculous life-saving procedure. To be successful, it required major pre-planning and the cohesive handing off from one trained specialist to the next. In all, it took orthopedists, neurosurgeons, vascular surgeons, internists, plastic surgeons, and a slew of specially trained surgical nurses to complete the nearly thirty-six-hour marathon surgery.

Once finished, it was declared a success. The two young twins would now be able to live a normal life. *Wow, amazing,* and *incredible* would be appropriate superlatives. I do believe that surgery and its outcome was a miracle. I remember watching and thinking, "That's what medicine is for."

Unfortunately, as we roll through this chapter, you will find out that the miracle of the Siamese twin operation was the exception and not the rule in medicine. It is true that in emergency situations and in specialty surgeries like the one I just described, modern medicine is phenomenal. As a matter of fact, the United States has the best crisis care in the world, bar none. But the harsh reality is that when it comes to managing your health and trying to bring you back from chronic sickness and disease, "modern medicine" is so far behind the times it's not even funny. Actually, the term *modern medicine* is a complete oxymoron; many of the medical procedures used today in the diagnosis and treatment of numerous health conditions are no different than in 1955. The only thing that has changed is the name of the drugs. That could hardly be described as *modern.* Wouldn't you agree?

I know I'm coming out swinging here, but if you ever want to achieve optimal health and performance in your life, this is a topic you will have to thoroughly grasp. Let's examine this a little closer.

The Difference in Mind-Set between
Healthy versus Unhealthy People

Before I get into statistics, I'd like to talk to you about the difference in mindset between people who live optimally healthy lives and those who lead unhealthy lives.

In all my years of teaching about health, either from a stage or via the written word, it has been my experience that people get as emotional talking about their beliefs in health as they do talking about religion or politics. As you'll discover in future chapters, creating genuine health means doing things that most people aren't used to doing. I have seen people in my audiences get worked into a frenzy over the differences between what needs to be done to be healthy and what they previously believed to be the best ways to take care of their health. What I'm about to say is of the utmost importance. *If you truly want to create amazing health in your body, you have to have a mind that is open and willing to accept new information that may go against everything you've ever believed about health.*

I may as well come right out and hit you with one of the hardest concepts to internalize. In a truly healthy body, there is no place for drugs. As a matter of fact, drugs and health are complete and total polar opposites. Now, don't get me wrong—I do understand and appreciate the need for medication in certain conditions. Many diabetics need insulin. Certainly there are heart patients and those with various neurological problems who need drugs. When my son got pneumonia, I was glad to have antibiotics for him. You get the picture, right? I'm not some crazy zealot who believes that there is never a time for medicine, but the point is, way-y-y too many people are taking drugs, both prescription and over-the-counter (OTC), that they absolutely do not need. That being said, if you are currently on prescription drugs, don't just quit taking them without first consulting with your doctor. (I'll expand on this more in chapter 3.) If you truly want to change your life and create an incredible state of health, you must adopt a mindset that you will only use drugs as a last resort. Your goal should be to take as little medication as possible, preferably none, for your entire life.

Even when my family was going through our mold problem, we never took medicine, though several different types were offered to us. The average person will accept these medications without hesitation, thinking that if the doctor prescribed them, they must be of value. In many cases, this is not so. There are no drugs that would have helped our mold-related problems, and I knew that they would further complicate our situation. If you want to develop the mindset of an incredibly healthy person, you must start to question what you put into your body.

Having a mindset of health means just that. You must live your life with the intention of always having and creating good health. One thing I notice in many of my chronic-condition patients is that they seem to ask the question, "Why me?" This may come off the wrong way, but hear me out. Why not you? Chronic conditions affect people by the millions, so why *not* you? While certain conditions may be rare, poor health is not. Far too many people have bought into this fallacy that their state of health is determined by genetics. It's not. Remember this; if you are not doing things to purposely create good health in your life, poor health *will* find you.

I don't want to delve too deeply into the mindset issue just yet; I will discuss it in more detail in the next chapter. The point is, as you head into this book, I want you to realize that very few people maintain good health as a matter of luck. There are rules that healthy people follow, and it all starts with how they view their health. If you are someone who already follows a healthy lifestyle and you are still having health challenges, I have great news for you: I promise that as I continue, I will explain why you are having problems that nobody else has been able to figure out.

How Does the Health of Americans Stack Up to the Rest of the World?

I must warn you, the next several pages of this book may be very alarming to you. You will almost certainly learn things that you have never heard before, and I dare say that some of them will totally blow you away.

While I was an undergraduate studying pre-med courses, I first learned the term *iatrogenic death*. If you haven't heard this term before, it's important that you become familiar with it. *Iatrogenic death* means death caused by a medical procedure.

While researching medical errors, I found the following chart. It comes from the work of Dr. Carolyn Dean. Dr. Dean is an M.D. N.D. and wrote the book Death by Modern Medicine. She has given me permission to use it here. Even as a chiropractic physician, I was astonished the first time I saw these statistics. After speaking about these numbers in hundreds of seminars and workshops over the years, I am still amazed. If you don't find this subject shocking and disturbing, you are probably not paying enough attention. This chart makes the case nice and succinct. It lists various types of iatrogenic death; along with how much money such errors cost our economy each year.

Condition	Deaths	Cost	Author
Adverse Drug Reactions	106,000	$12 billion	Lazarou Suh
Medical Error	195,000	$2.85 billion	Health Grades
Bedsores	115,000	$55 billion	Xakellis Barczak
Infection	99,000	$5 billion	CDC
Malnutrition	108,800	--------	Nurses Coalition
Outpatients	199,000	$77 billion	Starfield Weingart
Unnecessary Procedures	37,136	$122,000	HCUP
Surgery-Related	32,000	$9 billion	AHRQ
TOTAL	**895,936**	**$282.85 billion**	

I want to point out a few very important items on this chart. First of all, it should really jump off the page at you that approximately 37,136 people die each year from **unnecessary procedures**. That means that nearly 40,000 people die each year from medical procedures that should never have been performed! That is insane! What if that was your child or one of your parents? What if it was you? I am frequently shocked in my practice to see how quickly most people will go under the knife. A forty-eight-year-old male patient recently came into my office who has had several major surgeries that he absolutely did not need. He never even considered alternative options. As a matter of fact, I guarantee you I could have easily helped him correct those problems without surgery. His surgeries have left him with chronic problems that will only worsen as he ages. Even so-called "routine" surgeries are dangerous. This is not a game! This is your life!

Secondly, according to this chart, 106,000 people died from adverse drug reactions. Many other sources report this number is very conservative; some state that there are as many as around 250,000 deaths each year from adverse drug reactions. This should make you think twice when you take prescription drugs. All drugs are toxic chemicals and should not be taken lightly. When I was sick with mold poisoning I was having a difficult time breathing, so I went to an urgent care center. The doctor prescribed Advair. I got home and read the side-effects label. One of the first warnings on the label was increased chance of death. I threw it away. Not for me. I often find that the medications many of my patients have been taking for years are the root cause of the problems they suffer from. That is no exaggeration.

If you knew someone who used cocaine every day, you would expect that person to start suffering negative health effects, wouldn't you? As we all know, cocaine is a toxic chemical. Well, guess what? Prescription drugs and over-the-counter drugs are toxic chemicals too. So why wouldn't you expect that they would cause negative health effects, as cocaine does? I'll tell you why: that soothing voice at the end of drug commercials that so pleasantly describes the "rare but serious" side effects that may occur from taking said medication. The soothing voice makes it sound as though it would be an extreme rarity for one of those "side effects" to occur. Here's the thing. They aren't side effects; they're just effects. Read the side-effects label on the drugs that you take; that's what they are causing in your body. Maybe you're not experiencing all of them right now, but they are on the way.

The last point I want to make in regards to this chart is the total number of deaths. If you research the leading causes of death in the United States, the Center for Disease Control and the *Journal of the American Medical Association* will list heart disease as the number one cause of death and cancer as the number two cause of death. Let's look at these in a statistical format:

Heart Disease:	annual deaths—approximately **699,000**
Cancer:	annual deaths—approximately **560,000**
Medical Errors:	annual deaths—approximately **896,000**

You can clearly see that medical errors are the number one leading cause of death in our country. However, because all the various categories of iatrogenic death have to be added to arrive at this total, if you were to Google this statistic you would never find it.

This has been common knowledge to me for over a decade now and is the primary reason that my family uses medicine only as a last resort. When I say that we use it only as a last resort, I mean it.

Shortly after we moved to Virginia, my wife was hosting a woman's group at our house. One of the women approached her and asked if she could have a Tylenol because she had a headache. Wendy responded, "Sorry, we don't have any." The woman then said, "Well, how about an aspirin?" Wendy's response was, "No, we don't have any of that either. We don't keep any drugs in the house." The woman looked at my wife in disbelief and said, "Well, what do you do when one of you gets a headache?" Wendy replied, "We don't … ever." This statement was met with another look of disbelief.

Because we live a drug-free life, this reaction is something we have gotten used to. The reality is that the great majority of Americans keep a supply of over-the-counter drugs in their house large enough to make Walgreen's envious. Due to the trust that the American people have in medicine, most never give taking medication a second thought, but they should.

NSAIDS

The group of drugs that are most commonly abused by people are non-steroidal anti-inflammatory drugs (NSAIDS): over-the-counter painkillers. Let's consider Tylenol for a moment. This seems to be a drug of choice for many people for all kinds of issues, ranging from headaches to back pain. The following statement might surprise you.

A thousand capsules of Tylenol in a lifetime doubles the risk of end-stage renal disease.
(*New England Journal of Medicine*)

The above statement about how damaging this drug is to the kidneys comes from one of the most prestigious medical journals in the world. I heard a doctor state that Tylenol itself is the leading cause of kidney failure in our country. I don't know if that is true, but I wouldn't doubt it. You might be thinking, "Well, gosh, I would never use a thousand capsules of Tylenol in my life." Really? I see patients every day who write on their paperwork that they have been taking four Tylenol a day, every day, for over a year. If you do the math, the total is 1460 capsules … in one year! If you want to achieve optimal health in your life, you must accept that constant over-the-counter drugging of your body is killing you. I mean that literally.

If I asked you to guess for which condition most people take over-the-counter painkillers, you might answer headaches or low back pain. Let me use those conditions to show you a prime example of how people get on the treadmill of bad health by taking these drugs.

Suppose you get a headache one day and decide to take Tylenol to give you some relief. You take two Tylenol, and within a couple of hours your headache is gone. The next day you get another headache, but it's mild, so you decide to ride it out. It goes away. A few days later, you get another headache, so you take two Tylenol, and it goes away. Now something different happens. The next day you get another headache, but this time instead of riding it out, you take Tylenol for the second day in a row. Your headache goes away, but the next day you get another pretty bad one, so you take some more Tylenol. There is now a vicious cycle going on in your body's chemistry that you aren't even aware of.

One of the main side effects of most over-the-counter painkillers is something called a *rebound headache*. Have you ever heard that term before? Most people haven't. What this means is that when you take the drug, the active ingredient dulls your nerve endings enough to create relief from the headache, but the next day you get another headache caused by the drug, pretty much a drug-induced hangover.

It is hard for most people in these situations to connect the dots, because all they know is that when they have a headache, the drug makes it go away.

Patients come to see me in my office that have been on this merry-go-round for literally years, even decades! Can you imagine? Many times, they will have been going to doctors with a headache problem for years, and none have ever attempted to help them identify what the real root cause of their problem was. The good news is that in most cases, just stopping the painkillers will dramatically decrease the number of headaches that these patients suffer from.

Now, let's look at people who might take painkillers for other conditions, such as upper or lower back pain. Again, suppose at the end of each day, you get burning pain between your shoulder blades. A friend tells you that she also gets upper back pain, and taking painkiller XYZ seems to help. So you try it, and your pain goes away. Yay! Not so fast—the next day, your upper back starts to hurt again. So you take the drug XYZ again, and again, your pain goes away. The next day, not only does your upper back start to hurt again, but you get a headache too. Drug XYZ is causing rebound headaches, and you are now dealing with two health conditions, when you only started out with one. Awesome!

This point illustrates how taking medication can offset your health and start you spinning in the wrong direction. The scenarios that I just described are not rare. They are very common, in fact. I see them in my patients regularly. Sadly, these examples are minor compared to most drug-related health problems. I am just scraping the surface here.

Blood Pressure and Cholesterol Hysteria

When going over patient files, I often find myself shaking my head over how many people are taking either blood pressure or cholesterol drugs. They often go hand in hand. In my opinion, these are two of the most needless and dangerous types of drugs out there. I do acknowledge that there are people who need these drugs, but in almost all cases, they should be used on a very short-term basis until the patient is able to actually fix the underlying cause of the problem. That hardly ever happens. Most patients I see who are on these drugs have been on them for years and have been told by their doctors that they will always be on them. Great plan!

First of all, as with most health problems, high blood pressure and high cholesterol are usually the result of poor lifestyle choices. Bad food, too much stress, and a sedentary lifestyle are the frequent culprits. Yes, I know some people take very good care of themselves and still have these types of problems, but they are rare. Also, I have met many people who think that they take good care of themselves, but what they think constitutes "good" really doesn't.

It is important to realize that cholesterol is a necessary part of normal physiological function in the human body. It is essential for the building of all cell membranes in the body and necessary for bile acid and sex hormone production. Considering how many men are on cholesterol-lowering drugs these days, it is no wonder that so many of them have problems with erectile dysfunction.

Why Does "Normal" Change?

Did you know that just about thirty years ago the upper level of normal cholesterol was 300? The normal level was changed to two hundred in the 1970s. Depending on which component of blood work you are looking at (i.e., hemoglobin, TSH, calcium, etc.) and what part of the country you are in, the accepted "normal" ranges can vary quite a bit from lab to lab—except one. Cholesterol is standardized at 200 at every single lab in America. Can you guess why? It's because cholesterol-lowering drugs are a billion-dollar business. These drugs fly off the shelves, and once you become a customer, you are pretty much a customer for life. And get this; I heard recently that they are trying to get the accepted "normal" for cholesterol lowered to 150! A hundred and fifty!

Here's the problem. I already mentioned that your cell membranes are made of cholesterol, but so are your nerves and your brain. If your brain is made of cholesterol and you take drugs that are designed to harm cholesterol, what do you think will happen to your brain? Also, since cholesterol is made in the liver and these drugs attack the production of cholesterol, what do you think will happen to the liver? As a matter of fact, in a surprising move, the FDA has just added new warnings about statin drugs causing memory loss and increased risk of type II diabetes. This is why so many people taking statin drugs are suffering severe, in many cases deadly, consequences.

So, has the human body evolved so much in the last thirty to forty years that our cholesterol numbers should have changed by nearly 150 points? That is ridiculous! This is a prime example of how medicine sometimes tries to outsmart the human body. Sadly, many of the decisions made about what is considered normal boils down to the projected sales and profits of pharmaceutical drugs. This kind of junk science motivated the former editor of one of the most prestigious medical journals in the world to make the following statement:

> """It is simply no longer possible to believe much of the clinical research that is published, or to rely on the judgment of trusted physicians or authoritative medical guidelines. I take no pleasure in this conclusion, which I reached slowly and reluctantly over my two decades as an editor of The New England Journal of Medicine."

Marcia Angell MD

The human body is magnificent regarding it's ability to heal. Normal is normal and it shouldn't change.

A Prime Example of Why Americans Are So Sick!

Imagine you were at one of my seminars, and up on the stage I was holding a syringe. I explain to the audience that I had a mixture of aluminum, mercury, and formaldehyde (embalming fluid), among other things, in the syringe. Would you let me inject you with it? You'd probably say no. I hope you'd say no. I mean, for gosh sakes, those are highly toxic chemicals.

What I'm about to tell you may knock your socks off. Every fall, our country is subjected to one of the biggest and most mass-marketed legal scams of all time. Television commercials promote it; they promote it in malls, drug stores, churches, schools, and doctor's offices. Millions of dollars go into promoting one of the most ridiculous, nonsensical and health-harming scams you could possibly buy into. Have you figured out what I'm talking about yet? Of course I am referring to the annual flu shot fiasco that has gotten as out of control as a runaway train.

This annual ritual continues to further worsen the health of Americans. You will see in the next twenty to thirty years, as more and more people begin to suffer neurodegenerative diseases like Parkinson's and Alzheimer's, the burden that will result from this farce. I'm telling you straight up, getting a flu shot is one of the most worthless and damaging things you could do to your body. Consider the following research by Dr. Hugh Fudenberg, MD.

Dr. Fudenberg lists the harmful ingredients present in a flu shot.

Thimerosal (Mercury/preservative)

Aluminum (additive)

Benzethonium chloride (antiseptic)

Methylparaben (antifungal)

Formaldehyde (disinfectant)

Ethylene glycol (antifreeze/deadly poison)

Phenol (disinfectant)

Dr. Fudenberg wrote a very detailed research study on this topic. The most startling of his conclusions included the neurological damage that one can expect to incur from taking the flu shot. He states, "If a person has had five consecutive flu shots, their chance of contracting Alzheimer's disease is ten times higher."

So basically he is saying that the chemicals in the flu vaccine are so toxic that they will begin to annihilate your central nervous system and brain so badly that you will eventually wind up in a nursing home because you are urinating all over yourself and forgetting your own name. Consider this too: Before Dr. Fudenburg began speaking out against the harmful ingredients in vaccines he was heralded as one of the great medical researchers. He had over 800 papers in peer review medical literature and was a leading immunologist. After he spoke out against these harmful drugs, the medical establishment took his license away and branded him a crazy man. That's what goes on behind the scenes. Am I being too harsh? I don't think so.

To be completely accurate, the above quote by Dr. Fudenberg was referring to vaccinations given between 1970 and 1980. I was part of a debate on the Internet with a pharmacist who said that if the flu shot really had mercury in it that the FDA would never approve it. In response, one of the other doctors included in the debate produced the following link to the Center for Disease Control website listing the flu shot ingredients.

http://www.cdc.gov/vaccines/pubs/pinkbook/downloads/appendices/b/excipient-table-2.pdf

I recommend you look up this link and examine this chart carefully. On the chart, find the squares that are named influenza. There are six of them. Four out of the six have the word thimerosal listed in the ingredients. Thimerosal is the industrial name for mercury. That alone is enough for me. You'll have to judge for yourself, but I'd rather get the flu and be sick for a few days than have mercury injected into me.

As I write this book, I am forty-two years old. When I was growing up, the flu was basically just a bad cold. I know when I make that statement to audiences, most agree that it was just a bad cold. Now, somehow, mass media and mass hysteria have managed to scare everyone into thinking that if you get the flu, you're going to die. By repeating these scare tactics year in and year out, Big Pharma has now racked up a huge supply of customers who will line up annually to have themselves and their children injected with these toxic chemicals. I believe these are crimes against humanity, and something needs to be done about it.

Ironically, a large portion of people who receive the flu shot every year still wind up getting the flu. Furthermore, many research articles say that since it is impossible to match the flu vaccine with each year's flu strain, you are really no more protected from the flu than those who are not vaccinated. I'd say "no duh," but that sounds childish, right?

The Politics of Managed Care and Big Pharma

The above discussion about cholesterol drugs can be very shocking to some people. Many people believe that if the drugs were really dangerous, the FDA would not approve them. Have you ever heard of Vioxx, Seldane, and Fen-Phen? These are drugs that were approved by the FDA that killed tens of thousands of people before they were removed from the market. Watch late-night television and you will see several different commercials for class action lawsuits against drugs that are killing and maiming people—all of which were approved by the FDA! Let me make one thing very clear. Just because the FDA approves something, does not in any way mean that it is safe. There are prime examples of this popping up all over the place. Consider this quote from an article in Natural News:

Those of us who have long been describing the pharmaceutical industry as a "criminal racket" over the last few years have been wholly vindicated by recent news. Drug and vaccine manufacturer Merck was caught red-handed by two of its own scientists faking vaccine efficacy data by spiking blood samples with animal antibodies. GlaxoSmithKline has just been fined a whopping $3 billion for bribing doctors, lying to the FDA, hiding clinical trial data and fraudulent marketing. Pfizer, meanwhile has been sued by the nation's pharmacy retailers for what is alleged as an "overarching anticompetitive scheme" to keep generic cholesterol drugs off the market and thereby boost its own profits.

You can read this entire article at: http://www.naturalnews.com/036417_glaxo_merck_fraud.html#ixzz20CduuNLp

The American Medical Association, the FDA, the pharmaceutical companies, and managed care companies coexist in peaceful harmony. This is the reason why you hear so many negative things about natural and alternative forms of healthcare from the conventional medical profession.

It still amazes me how frequently I hear, "My medical doctor says I should never get adjusted by a chiropractor," or "My doctor doesn't believe in chiropractic." Really? There is a plethora of solid scientific research in the medical literature to back up the safety and effectiveness of chiropractic. This has been true for decades, yet people still espouse such nonsense. What it boils down to is that every dollar spent in an alternative healthcare setting is a dollar taken away from the bottom line of the medical industry.

Currently, the FDA is trying to gain control of the vitamin and supplement industry. If you take vitamins on a regular basis, you will notice on any packaging a statement that reads something to the effect of, "These statements have not been evaluated by the FDA." The FDA hasn't regulated vitamins because they believed that supplements didn't do anything to change health conditions. Supposedly, only drugs could do that. Now there is a voluminous body of research proving how beneficial vitamins are. The supplement industry is a billion-dollar industry, and the FDA wants it. All of it. If they were to gain control, you would literally have to go to your medical doctor and get a prescription just to get some vitamin C or a multivitamin. Ridiculous? That's your trusty FDA in action.

As doctors, shouldn't our job be to do what is best for the patients that we serve? I am strongly against drugs and surgery, but even I recognize their time and place, and I do refer patients to the appropriate treating specialty when necessary because I want what is best for my patients. Do I believe that I deserve to make a nice living? You bet I do. I spent eight years and a hell of a lot of money on an education so I could help people lead better lives. But I would never endorse anything in my clinic or my teachings at the expense of a patient's best interest just to make a buck.

To be clear, I am not suggesting that people who work in the medical field are bad people. Not even close. I personally know many people who work in medicine, and they are the finest of people, with the best intentions. The problem lies in the organizations that run medicine, and it has been that way for decades. So much so that many people who work in medicine are indoctrinated with this "drug only, no alternative healthcare" thinking in school. The AMA and FDA are smart. They know that if they indoctrinate practitioners in school, they can continue to perpetuate this stupid game forever.

I once had a young female come to me who was suffering from migraine headaches and had been for years. I knew that I could help her. However, her husband was a medical doctor, and he would not let her come to my office. He actually told me that he was taught in medical school not to work with chiropractors. He proudly told me that he would continue to treat his wife with drug therapy, which she had already been doing for quite some time to no avail. That was four years ago. I know I could have helped her, and I hope for her sake that she is better, but I seriously doubt it. Tragic.

How would you feel if you were the patient of that doctor and you had a condition that could best be served by chiropractic care and he didn't tell you that? Instead, he prescribed a drug for you that didn't work and will cause future health problems in the form of side effects. Sadly, as this doctor's patient, while he stands smiling in front of you, you will most likely never know that he has done you a tremendous disservice.

Reality Check

I have a clear and distinct purpose for this chapter, and I am not afraid to say what it is. As I illustrated with the story of the Siamese twins in the opening paragraph of this chapter, modern medicine can do some incredibly powerful and beneficial things, given the right situation. But I want to unleash a shock-and-awe campaign about the current state of medicine in our society. I feel it is necessary to shake the foundations of many people who are in dire need of help. If people don't understand the reality, then they may never have a chance to get well. I hope at the very least I dropped some bombs that opened your eyes to a new vision.

In my second year of practice I had a female patient come to see me for lower back pain. She was in her late thirties. Before entering the exam room to meet with her, I looked over her file. She was severely overweight, smoked a pack of cigarettes a day, was on medication for high blood pressure and high cholesterol, and had both her gallbladder and part of her colon removed. Her occupation was receptionist at the prestigious Mayo Clinic, which was just a few miles from my office.

As I began my consultation with her, I asked leading questions about her health to help me best determine the course of action to take with her. In the middle of my questioning, she stopped me and said, "Doc, other than this lower back pain, I'm healthy as a horse!" I was very taken aback by this and literally laughed out loud. I asked her "Who told you that?" She responded by proudly saying, "My doctors at the Mayo Clinic."

This overweight smoker had had organs removed and was taking drugs for high blood pressure and high cholesterol. Does that sound like healthy to you? Me neither. But all of her blood work at the time was normal, and she didn't have any signs of apparent disease, so by medical standards, she was healthy. And that, my friends, sums up this entire chapter.

If you truly wish to achieve a level of optimal health in your life, you must realize that drugs and surgery will most likely not get you there. You need to develop a mindset that you will go the extra mile to create health in your life. This means you will put in the time to learn and do things that promote health and eliminate those things that lower your health potential. It's time you took control of your life!

Chapter 3

Fixing Chronically Bad Health

All disease is reversible.
There is no such thing as a terminal condition.
Only terminal treatments and terminal mindsets.

—Aiya

If there was one underlying theme that I hope you got out of chapter 1, it's the fact that when it comes to suffering from chronic health problems, I genuinely know how you feel. I believe that everything in life happens for a reason, and the reason that my family had to go through that mold situation was so that I could better help people who are suffering from chronically bad health.

Nothing prepares you more for understanding any situation in life than having been there yourself, and, boy, have I been there. As I already said, I understand the frustration. I get it! In this chapter, I'm going to show you why nobody has yet been able to help you and what you need to do to turn your life around.

Hammers and Nails

Since I will be talking a lot about chronic health problems, I would like to give you my definition of what a chronic health problem is. In my office, we define any problem that's been ongoing for more than three months as chronic. If you have been having migraine headaches once or twice a week, every week, for longer than three months, in my mind, you have a chronic problem. If you have had acid reflux burning in your chest several times a week, every week, for longer than three months, you have a chronic health problem. If you have been chronically fatigued the majority of the week, every week, for longer than three months, you have a chronic health problem.

So let's examine what got you to where you are at, which I assume is the reason you are reading this book. You fall under one of two categories. You are either someone who is simply interested in improving your overall level of health or you are someone in dire straits and need a complete health overhaul. No matter which category you are in, understanding this chapter is critical for your future health.

One thing I hope was glaringly obvious to you in chapter 2 is that the paradigm of healthcare we have in our society is totally broken. Furthermore, following that path of healthcare will lead you to poor health and possibly even early death, as it did with my mother.

If you have chronically bad health, or you think you feel good but you take several medications every day to achieve that, listen up. There is a saying I like that really helps to illustrate what happens when most people visit the doctor, and it goes like this: When you are a hammer, all you see is nails. Translation: you only see one thing. If we apply this saying to healthcare, it means that when you go to a doctor for help, they see only one type of treatment, and it's drugs. If you go to your doctor with fibromyalgia, they see Lyrica. If you go to your doctor with a thyroid problem, they see Synthroid. If you go to your doctor with back pain, they see Flexoril. I can hear the medical professionals protesting about what I just said. How can they argue that point? If you walk into your doctor's office with one of those problems, you are going to walk out with a prescription. That's just how it works.

To be fair, many natural health practitioners are also hammers seeing nails. You go to a chiropractor with fibromyalgia; he or she adjusts your spine. You go to an acupuncturist with a thyroid problem; he or she works on the meridians that control the thyroid gland. It's all one-track-mind thinking. Unfortunately, the body doesn't work that way.

Many times I will have patients come listen to my lectures. Then they want to take what I teach them and ask their medical doctor's opinion of it. If that is what you are planning on doing after reading this book, let me save you the trip. Your medical doctor will not accept what I teach you in this book. I promise you that.

The concepts and ideas presented here are very progressive. If your doctor was in agreement with or even aware of them, you wouldn't still be suffering. You will have to make the decision about whether you want to continue down the same path you have always taken or whether you want to really take charge of your health. It's up to you. That's not to say that if you're under medical care for a condition that you just stop taking your meds or quit going to treatment. In some cases, you must co-manage your care between your natural healthcare provider and your medical doctor. Common sense usually wins out.

But if you are trying to reach the upper limits of good health or are trying to get past a chronic health problem, you need a progressive doctor who isn't just a hammer seeing nails.

You Aren't Reading This Just Because ...

I hold workshops in my office that pertain to certain types of chronic conditions, such as fibromyalgia, sciatica, migraine headaches, peripheral neuropathy, vertigo, biotoxic disorders and weight loss. One thing I tell people in my workshops is that they are not there just because they have fibromyalgia or migraine headaches. It's not that simple.

There are more likely than not numerous neurological and metabolic issues going on in your body that are at the root of your named diagnosis. Let me show you what I mean.

Neurological

If you experience even a few of the following symptoms, you have some sort of neurological dysfunction going on:

- Loss of short term memory

- Balance problems

- Problems concentrating

- Noticing that your handwriting is getting worse

- Numbness or tingling in your hands or feet

- Headaches

- Ringing in the ears

- Increased sensitivity to sunlight

- Getting lost in conversation

Don't worry; this isn't something you need to run to the emergency room for. I'm not talking about disease or pathology here, but your brain just isn't functioning the way that it should. From a functional neurology perspective, you have a frequency of firing issue somewhere in your brain. It could be in the temporal lobe, parietal lobe, frontal cortex, cerebellum, or some other area of the brain. You could have issues in multiple areas. The only way to find out is through proper neurological analysis. These problems could be manifesting as a whole host of health challenges.

An untold number of people experiencing these kinds of problems are not receiving proper treatment for their condition. For example, if someone has decreased firing in the right side of their brain, one of the possible outcomes could be muscle twitching or tremors. Treated according to the medical model, this patient would probably be given drugs ranging from Neurontin to anxiety pills, muscle relaxers, or levodopa, the drug of choice for Parkinson's. It matters not which drug is given; it will never, ever fix the problem. As a matter of fact, treating this way will ensure that the patient's condition will worsen over time, because drugs will not fix the problem in the brain that is causing symptoms.

Conversely, when treated with functional neurology, the patient has a much greater chance for success. I have a fifty-one-year-old female patient who had continuous, terrible tremors in her left arm that had been going on for years. I performed a simple functional rehab therapy on her with a cloth device known as optokinetic tape, or OPK. The OPK is roughly thirty inches long and has alternating red and white squares on it. The doctor holds the OPK in front of the patient and has the patient track the red squares with their eyes as he moves it in different patterns. This process helps to establish a more normal firing sequence in the brain. I did this OPK therapy on my patient upon her first visit in my office. It literally took less than one minute before her tremor stopped. My patient was quite astonished, to say the least. The tremor returned in about a month. When she came back, I performed the therapy during three more sessions, and months later she still has no tremor. That is how you create healing!

Most people are being medicated for such types of functional problems; they should be undergoing functional neurological rehabilitation. Many of these problems develop from metabolic conditions elsewhere in the body, which is what we will cover next.

Metabolic Problems

Just as it was important to discuss neurological problems, it is equally important to discuss metabolic factors.

Blood Sugar

Because approximately 35 percent of the American population is overweight and a high percentage of those people are on a collision course towards diabetes, blood sugar can be a real doozy! From a functional medicine viewpoint, your blood sugar should reside somewhere in the neighborhood between eighty-five and ninety-nine on a serum glucose test for you to be healthy. If your blood sugar is lower than eighty-five, you may suffer from hypoglycemia or reactive hypoglycemia, both of which can cause major problems in your energy levels and your body's ability to heal.

More commonly, most people's blood sugar exceeds the preferred high of ninety-nine. If your level is above this, you may be insulin resistant, have metabolic syndrome (pre-diabetes), or be moving full-steam ahead toward type II diabetes. We are talking about serious business here, so I hope you're paying attention. If your fasting blood glucose level is over ninety-nine, you need to start working hard to bring it down. Failing to do so will lead to an extremely poor state of health and possibly early death. In chapter 6, I will teach you how to clean up your blood sugar. Don't worry—we'll get you there.

If you experience some of the following symptoms, you may have blood sugar issues that need to be dealt with:

- Craving sweets throughout the day

- Needing coffee to keep yourself going

- Feeling shaky or jittery

- Frequent urination

- Becoming irritable if a meal is skipped

- Fatigue that is relieved by eating

- Craving sweets after meals

- Difficulty losing weight

Adrenal Glands

I'd bet a large sum of money that after you read the next couple of paragraphs, you will be shaking your head in disbelief that no other doctor has discussed this with you before. These tiny little suckers can cause a world of problems for you.

Your adrenal glands, your stress glands, are two walnut sized glands that sit atop your kidneys. I won't go into the exact physiology, but when stressed, they begin to disrupt the proper function of cortisol, the stress hormone. It always amazes me how many patients come to me with a plethora of health problems and then tell me they have no stress. If your body is unhealthy, you have stress. This is such a serious issue that I devote an entire chapter to it in part two of this book.

When your adrenals are stressed, they start to dump cortisol. Cortisol does four really nasty things to you.

1. It attacks the hippocampus in your brain, which is responsible for your short-term memory. This is why you walk into a room and forget why you did so, and you frequently can't remember where you put your keys. It's not because you are getting old!

2. It affects your sleep cycles, either getting to sleep or staying asleep, or both. Sound familiar?

3. It causes pain cycles in your weakest areas. For example, if you are a person that suffers from lower back pain, it could attack the nerves in your lower back. This means that you could have the best chiropractor in the world, giving you the best adjustments in the world, and your back will still hurt.

4. It will trigger fat-storing hormones and either cause you to gain weight or have a very difficult time losing weight.

Let's recap: memory loss, trouble sleeping, pain, and weight gain. If you have chronic health problems, I probably just painted a picture of your life, and this gland has likely never been discussed with you before. I review a lot of medical records from my patients and it's rare that they have had their adrenal glands checked prior to coming to my office.

You may have adrenal problems if you have some of the following symptoms:

- Difficulty falling asleep

- Difficulty staying asleep through the night

- Getting fatigued in the afternoon

- Have difficulty getting going in the morning

- Frequent cravings for salty foods

- Weak or brittle fingernails

- Chronic fatigue

Stomach

A couple of very common health challenges in present-day society arise out of the stomach. One condition is known as hypochlorhydria. This is a condition where the stomach does not produce enough stomach acid, which can lead to several problems related to the digestion of food and can cause gas, bloating, and bad breath. Those three symptoms will send people to the drugstore in droves to get their hands on over-the-counter medications. Hypochlorhydria can also lead to bacterial and parasitic infections and eventually cause vitamin deficiencies in the body.

When stomach acid production is low, food, especially protein, will sit in your stomach and begin to become rancid and putrefied. The rotten food sitting in your gut can actually cause burning and acid reflux–like symptoms in your esophagus and chest. Then when you go to your doctor and inform her of your symptoms, she will tell you that you have gastroesophageal reflux disease (GERD) and then prescribe a drug that is designed to reduce your stomach acid! This means you will have less acid than you already do, increasing your problems with hypochlorhydria, and your body will be getting sicker and sicker. Don't you think it would actually make more sense to try and fix the problem than to just make it worse by medicating the symptoms?

The second condition related to the stomach is actually an excess of stomach acid. That doesn't mean that if you have acid reflux symptoms you should just go and get a prescription. I ask my patients who are on drugs like Protonix or Prilosec, "How long do you plan on being on this drug?" Most people will sit dumbfounded when asked this question, because it is usually at that point when they realize their only plan is to be on the drug for the rest of their life. That is not a good plan. Again, don't you think it would be smarter to actually try and fix the cause of the problem? Remember, to develop a mindset of natural health, you should think about drugs only as a last resort.

There may be problems with your stomach if you experience some of the following:

- Sense of fullness during or after meals

- Frequent use of antacids

- Frequent heartburn

- Indigestion

- Acid reflux

- Belching, burping or bloating

- Difficult bowel movements

- Chronically bad breath

What Is Normal?

If you're wondering why your medical doctor has never warned you about these issues while reviewing your blood work, let me explain. The upper- and lower-end ranges of normal on medical labs are pathological. What that means is that by the time a particular lab value on a blood panel falls outside of that range, you may be in trouble. Most likely your body has been dealing with that particular problem for a long time. Let me give you an example.

The component of your blood work used to evaluate the thyroid gland is called TSH (thyroid stimulating hormone). In medical labs, "normal" TSH numbers are anywhere between .45 and 4.56. That is an incredibly wide range. You won't be diagnosed with hypothyroidism until you pass the upper range of 4.56. In functional medicine, we use lab ranges that were compiled by the American Academy of Clinical Chemists based on healthy people. On a functional scale of healthy people, a normal TSH range is between 1.8 and 3.0. That range is obviously much tighter. If you have a TSH number of 4.25, you haven't officially exceeded the upper number of 4.56, but something in your thyroid physiology is not working correctly. Does that make sense? In chart format, this is what it would look like:

.45	.46 to 1.7	1.8 to 3.0	3.1 to 4.55	4.56
Abnormally low level on medical labs	Considered normal but is not	Normal TSH for healthy people	Considered normal but is not	Abnormally high level on medical labs

This is why you can have all kinds of problems, and doctors continue to review your blood work and tell you everything is normal. I know this has happened to you. When I was going through my mold problem, it happened to me about ten times!

Here's the point I want you to take away from this section: you probably have numerous systems in your body that are not functioning properly, and they are at the root of your chronic health problems. I don't care what your problem is. It doesn't matter if you suffer from migraine headaches, chronic fatigue, carpel tunnel syndrome, or even autoimmune problems like lupus, Crohn's disease or Hashimoto's thyroiditis. If you fix these systems in your body, you will improve! You may not cure your disease or health condition, but you'll have more good days than bad, and you'll feel better than you have in ages.

The Unhealthy➔Symptom➔Drug Paradox

Are you wondering why your primary care physician or specialist has never explained all this to you? It all goes back to hammers seeing nails. The topics discussed in the previous paragraphs do not fit into the drug treatment paradigm. Nor do they fit into a treatment program that is based on what health insurance will pay for. Ours is a tragically broken healthcare system based on an outdated philosophy of healthcare.

I want to take some of the problems talked about above and apply them to how they would play out in a real-life setting. Follow me on this. At some point in your life, one of your body's systems begins to fail. The reason it fails is prolonged exposure to various stresses and strains that you are exposed to throughout your life. When I say that one of your body's systems begins to fail, in essence I am saying that a particular part of your body becomes unhealthy. When it becomes unhealthy it starts to produce a symptom. Let's say that symptom is migraine headaches. You go to your primary care physician with migraine headaches and he says, "No problem. We have Imitrex, we've got Percocet. Heck, we're even giving Botox injections for that." Now, you are managing the symptoms of migraine headaches with drugs. Your symptoms might improve, but was the problem causing the symptom fixed? No! So what are you left with? You are still unhealthy, which is why the migraines started in the first place.

I know these next few paragraphs may seem redundant, but follow me on this because I'm going to make a big point here. Now you are taking Imitrex for your migraine headache problem, but you are still unhealthy. Six months later, your body produces another symptom. Let's say it's acid reflux. Again, you go to your primary care physician and explain that after you eat, you get burning chest pain. Your doctor says, "Hey, no problem. We have Prilosec, Protonix, and Nexium.

We've got all kinds of drugs for that." Problem solved, right? Wrong! Your symptoms might be improved, but did the drug fix the problem causing the symptom? No! So what are you left with? You are still unhealthy, but now you are taking two different drugs to manage two different conditions.

A few months down the road, you begin to notice that you are becoming more and more fatigued. On a daily basis, you feel sluggish, and you are having a hard time getting everything done because you have no energy. Off you go again to your primary care physician. You explain that you have been feeling fatigued, and your doctor says, "Hey, no problem. I can prescribe Lyrica for that." All better, right? Wrong again! Maybe your fatigue is a little better now, although it's been my experience with patients that it won't be, but if it was, did it fix the problem causing the fatigue? No! So what are you left with? You are now taking three different drugs to manage three different conditions, and you are still unhealthy.

Just for fun, a couple of years into this process, the Imitrex that you have been taking for migraine headaches starts to cause a symptom, which we call a side effect. (I don't know why they call them side effects when they are in fact just effects. You take drugs, you get effects. There's no "side" about it.) Let's say this side effect is anxiety, which is one of the common so-called side effects of Imitrex. Once more you head to your primary care physician, explaining you just haven't been feeling right. You are anxious and seem nervous all the time. Your doctor is quick to inform you that he can prescribe Xanax, the drug of choice for anxiety. It is also one of the most overly prescribed, health-damaging drugs on the market. I actually believe this class of drugs to be a crime against humanity. Your doctor most likely will not even suggest that the Imitrex could be causing your anxiety. Instead of actually trying to figure out what is wrong with you, your doctor immediately prescribes another drug. I don't blame your doctor for this. I blame the whole philosophy of traditional medicine. As I have stated a couple of times already, medicine is great for acute crisis care, but when it come to managing your health, modern medicine is a broken and outdated philosophy of care.

Allow me to put this whole scenario into perspective. A couple of years into this process, you are now managing four different health conditions with four different drugs. Neither you nor your doctor has come one single itsy bitsy little step closer to actually fixing any of the reasons why your body began to break down in the first place. If you continue in this manner, you will very soon undoubtedly be taking even more drugs to manage the new conditions that will pop up in the future. At this point, what must you conclude? You must conclude that what you are doing is not working, and your doctor has no idea how to fix your problems!

The initial symptom I described in this cascade was migraine headaches. What would have happened if your doctor had figured out what was at the root of those migraines and fixed it, rather than just prescribing a drug to manage the symptoms? More likely than not, your doctor would have discovered that your migraines were being caused by either a structural problem in your neck, a food sensitivity or a biotoxin. Figuring that out and applying the appropriate treatment, none of which would require drugs, would save you from a downhill slide in the future. Addressing your neck, food sensitivity or ridding your body of biotoxins would prevent you from a lifetime of bad health. Do you see how much more effective that would be than just drugging each symptom that pops up?

I witness similar scenarios in my practice all the time. Patients come in who are on a plethora of drugs, and some of them are now dealing with so many different conditions that they can't even remember what started it all in the first place. *You cannot poison a body into good health!*

Often in such situations as I am going over a patient's chart and I notice they are taking a dozen medications or more, I will think to myself, "If this person can just see through the haze, I could change her life." Unfortunately, sometimes patients cannot see through the haze. Many of them believe so strongly in their medication and the medical profession that their judgment is clouded. The reality is that medications are doing nothing except altering the natural biochemistry of their body and screwing up different systems to the point that full recovery can be very difficult. People don't realize that their meds are damaging different tissues and cells, thus shortening their lifespan. As my good friend Dr. Andy Barlow says in his Mississippi accent, "All those drugs are doing is numbing ya and dumbing ya."

It can be frustrating as I review cases like these, because I know that if the patients could throw away all the medications, get back to baseline zero, and start over, our chance for success would be much greater. When bad health has entrenched itself in their life, a lot of people continue to go to their doctor blindly, never realizing that they are just medicating symptoms and not really getting to the root of their problem. This process continues to compound chronically bad health; as every day passes, the health of the individual involved continues to deteriorate.

What about Autoimmunity?

The amount of people suffering from autoimmune conditions has gotten out of control in the last decade. I know that in my practice, the numbers of people coming in now with autoimmune (AI) problems are dramatically increased compared to my first few years.

We have always been told that AI problems are genetic and that there is pretty much nothing you can do about them, except to medicate, manage, and hope for the best. Well, in functional medicine we know that not to be true.

First of all, very few problems that people deal with are the results of a poor genetic makeup. It certainly is easier to blame AI problems on genetics, but we now know that most of these conditions are actually caused by epigenetics, which are environmental factors. To boil it all the way down, AI problems result from those things we do to ourselves, and the things that we are exposed to in our environment. I am not saying that genetics don't matter and I will explain how they come into play in a moment.

If that all sounds pretty radical to you, wait till you hear this. What if I told you that all autoimmune conditions are the same disease? Pretty radical thought right? Think about it. Lupus, Hashimoto's, Scleroderma, Multiple Sclerosis, Fibromyalgia, Sjogren's Syndrome,

Dermatomyositis, Ulcerative Colitis, the list goes on and on; all the same. You might ask, how can that be? Well, autoimmunity is autoimmunity. It is just manifested differently in each individual based upon his or her genetic blueprint. The epigenetic factors cause it, and the genetic makeup determines which disease it will be.

If you are someone who suffers from an autoimmune problem I can guarantee that there is one thing that has probably never been explained to you. There are two halves to your immune system. They are known as TH1 and TH2. They should stay in even balance with each other. When one side of the immune system becomes dominant, then you have autoimmunity. The reason that AI patients are told that nothing can be done to resolve their condition is because traditional medicine has never been able to resolve the factors that keep that particular half of the person's immune system in a dominant mode.

In functional medicine, we have great success dealing with these problems. The first thing we do is figure out whether the patient is TH1 or TH2 dominant. Once we do this we can immediately start supplementing the appropriate nutritional factors that support the weak side of the immune system and eliminate those things that trigger the dominance. Most patients will usually see an immediate improvement in symptoms just from doing this.

The next piece of the puzzle is to find out what is causing the imbalance in the first place. In other words, is it an active antigen such as a bacteria or virus? Is it a food sensitivity? Is it heavy metal toxicity or a bio toxin? These are all epigenetic factors that cause autoimmunity and there can definitely be more than one. Once we can identify and eliminate all possible factors that are causing the problems, in most cases the patient can go on to lead a normal life.

While I don't claim to be able to cure autoimmune disease, I know for sure that tremendous improvements can be made. For some people they can see their autoimmunity go dormant. For others, they can see massive improvement in their quality of life. One thing I always ask my autoimmune patients is, "what if we could even get you fifty percent better?" That is a very tantalizing thought to say the least.

Watching a person with an AI condition get tremendous improvement in their lives is one of the most gratifying parts of what I do. Most people suffering from these kinds of problems truly don't believe that there is any hope for them. If you go on the Internet and research some of these diseases, you will likely find all the dismal, gloom and doom research provided by the medical profession. Trust me, it does not have to be that way.

Getting Out of the Trap

What I hope you take away from this chapter is that the system of healthcare utilized in our society is not congruous with good health. For many people, it is like quicksand that they are sucked into. Unless someone comes and throws them a lifeline, they will surely continue to sink.

One of the bigger challenges lies in the fact that if you are stuck in a medical rut, as I have just described, society will be right there to assure you that you are doing the right thing. If you ask your siblings, parents, neighbors, or friends for advice on how to resolve a health issue, you will get a unanimous vote: go see your doctor. Why? Because most people do whatever is popular. It absolutely blows my mind how often I hear people talking about going to the doctor and being medicated for health issues without that doctor even bothering to find out what is at the root cause of their problem.

If you go against the grain, which is what you must do to overcome poor health, you will likely meet resistance. A female patient came to me recently with fibromyalgia and chronic abdominal pains. I put her on a program, and she began seeing phenomenal results. She even lost more than twenty pounds as an outcome of our treatment protocol. Her best friend tried talking her out of coming to see me, saying that she felt it was dangerous for her to be losing weight and taking natural supplements. Incredible! But that's what sometimes happens when you live a naturally health life.

In the first part of this book, I wanted to let you know that I understand firsthand what it is like to suffer from chronically poor health and that I know what it takes to fix it. I also wanted to show you how messed up and broken our medical system is. If you are mired in medical healthcare, your chances of achieving truly optimal health are slim to none.

Now that we've discussed sickness and what doesn't work, let's move into part two and work on getting you healthy!

PART II

Returning to Health

Chapter 4

Creating the Vision of a New You

Good health is the groundwork of all happiness.

—Leigh Hunt

In part one of this book, you learned about the dismal current reality of where our healthcare system is. As I stated in the first three chapters and really believe in my heart, it is absolutely necessary for you to understand how bad it is and how devastating it can be to your overall health to continuously go down that path of healthcare.

In part two of this book, we will address the solutions to poor health. This will be the "how-to": how to make your body healthier; how to overcome poor health; how to take your health to the next level; how to maintain excellent health for the rest of your life! In short, part two will be the nuts and bolts of good health.

Throughout the rest of this book I will give you both the tangibles and intangibles of how to improve your health, simple things to do that will make massive changes in your life. I will be blowing the lid off of all the stupid nutrition information that has been being taught in our country for the last few decades and teach you how to really fuel your body. I'll show you that you don't have to spend hours on end in a gym to obtain a healthy body. And I'm going to explain to you why you can't get a good night's sleep. That might sound like small potatoes, but improving just those three aspects of your life could conceivably regulate blood sugar, lower cholesterol, and improve adrenal function.

How do these systematic changes translate to real-life improvements? For starters, simply regulating your blood sugar could dramatically reduce pain in your body. Many people already know some of the things they need to do in order to achieve optimal health, but they won't do them. Will you? The answer to that question will have a significant impact on the rest of your life.

In addition, I will be addressing the all-too-important topic of how you identify with yourself and what your core beliefs are. We're going to work on some visualization techniques and solidify a new way to view your health. If you take massive action on what I teach you, when I'm done with you, you're going to be a new person. My goal is to give you all the tools you need for success and at the same time keep it simple.

Also, I will give you a list of action steps to work on at the end of each remaining chapter.

> # Take care of your body. It's the only place you have to live.

Fun, Fun, Fun!

Chapter 4 is going to be a fun chapter! In this chapter you get to create the ideal you—the you that you've always wanted to be. What could be better than that?

Frequently I hear people say, "I sure wish I was healthier," or "I need to regain my health." So I have a question for you. What does getting healthier, or regaining your health, mean to you? If you don't know what good health would mean to you, how will you know if you achieve it? For example, one person might consider achieving good health to mean getting his blood pressure under control and losing twenty pounds, while another person might think good health means having the energy to work out every day and throwing away their antidepressants. You have to be clear about what health means to you before you can achieve it.

One of the biggest challenges I see in people who are not healthy is their identification with being an unhealthy person. This goes back to telling their story, as I discussed in chapter 1. Such people cannot even picture themselves living a life of fantastic health. They don't believe it's possible for them, so they continue to identify with being an unhealthy person. If this is a problem for you, you *must* change that! You must begin to identify with being an incredibly healthy person. If you don't, you will continue to sabotage your health by living out the same bad habits that you always have.

I am going to do my best to get you to dig deep and really create the healthiest physical, mental, and emotional version of yourself that you've ever imagined. One of the reasons that many patients can't ever get well is because fundamentally they can't even visualize themselves being well. They don't even know what *well* means to them. They can't visualize what it would be like to be healthy and vital and to be able to walk on a beach without feeling out of breath or their joints aching or knowing that they will pay for it later. They can't imagine what it would be like to wear clothes that make them proud of the way they look in them. They can't visualize what it would be like to be able to go and do whatever they want to do and not wake up the next day riddled with pain. And many can't visualize living without popping twenty-five pills every day just to maintain a poor quality of life. They just can't visualize themselves having excellent health.

It starts there. It's worthless to even try to improve your health until you know what good health means to you. My sincere wish for you is that by the end of this chapter you will have a new and clear vision of what you would like to accomplish with your health. Ideally, you will be filled with hope, enthusiasm, and high expectations about what you can achieve.

Planning Your Own Death

Have you ever planned your own death? For a chapter that is supposed to be filled with fun and happiness, it doesn't sound very inspirational, does it? Think about it, though. How can you live a long, happy, healthy life to a ripe old age if you don't even know what age you want to live to? I know a lot of people will respond with some version of, "Well, that's completely out of my control," or "That's all up to God," or "That's all dependent on when I'm programmed to die."

While some of that may be true, my belief is that if you don't have an ideal vision of how long you'd like to live in good health, then you will just suffer the same miserable ending as most people do, and probably sooner than you should. For example, my goal or vision for myself is to live in a healthy, happy, and vital body until I'm a hundred years old. How can I ever make it there if I don't have a plan for that? Do you think that it's all based on good luck? If I don't focus on taking care of my body so that it will last me that long, my chances of making it there will be very, very slim.

Are there other life circumstances that could come along and change that for me? Could I get hit by a truck tomorrow and die? Possibly. Could I be the victim of a heinous crime and lose my life? Maybe. Could some other unforeseen health aberration or accident occur that takes my life earlier than I wanted? Of course. But I know that if my belief is that I want to live to a hundred years of age in a healthy body, then I can. I *strongly* believe that! And I know for a fact that believing in that gives me a better chance than if I don't.

That hundred-year vision is a beacon of light for me in times of challenge. When I was sick with mold poisoning, one of the major things that helped me get my life back was continuously reminding myself of my hundred-year goal. I remember saying to myself, "What I'm dealing with right now does not fit into my hundred-year plan. How can I get past this?" In my darkest days, when I felt like I might not live for another week, remembering my hundred-year goal gave me the strength and determination to keep moving back toward health. I truly believe it is one of the main reasons why today I am not only surviving but also thriving.

Many survivors of mold poisoning are told that they will most likely experience multiple chemical sensitivity (MCS) for the rest of their lives. Having MCS means that you are easily set off by all kinds of chemicals, including detergents, cologne, perfume, deodorants, cleaning supplies, hair gels—and the list goes on and on. When exposed to chemical irritants, the patient who suffers with MCS can experience respiratory distress, fatigue, pain, and myriad other symptoms. In my mind, I knew for a fact that MCS was not going to fit into my hundred-year plan. After all, I like wearing cologne, and I love smelling my wife's perfume. Should I just give in and be unable to enjoy those things? I literally told myself that there was no way I was going to buy into that. I refused to believe that I would be victim to that problem for the rest of my life. And you know what? I'm not.

What ripe old age would you like to live to in good health? At what age do you envision yourself being able to remain active with your kids and grandkids? At what age do you think you'll want to stop making love to your spouse? Have you ever thought about that? Until what age would you like to be able to travel the world in good health? These are critically important questions to ask yourself.

Both of my parents died in their early sixties, which was only two years into my father's retirement. They never got to enjoy their retirement. They didn't get to do all the things they wanted to do, and that's why I would say that they checked out early. My parents didn't have a plan for how long they wanted to live, and they treated their bodies accordingly. I know that if they had the opportunity, they would do things differently. I know that they would want more time with their grandkids, more time with each other—more time, period.

So how about it? It's time for you to start planning your death. Not in a literal way. I don't sit around dwelling on death or thinking about how I want to die or where I want to die or any of the morbid details. To me, what the term "planning your own death" means is that I know that I want to live until I'm one hundred years old. After that, I will be happily ready for eternity. That's my plan. It's time you started to make a plan too.

I'm going to ask you to choose a number. There is no wrong answer here. Whatever your number, that is the right one. Maybe you only want to live to be seventy. If that's the case, I'd suggest that maybe there are other areas of your life that you are not happy with. I mean, if you were living a fulfilled, fantastic, awesome life, why would you only want to live until seventy? I suggest that you pick at least eighty—although it is your life and you have to pick what is right for you. Just remember that when you are setting an age goal, set it with the idea that you will live to that age in good health and with ultimate vitality. One of the reasons many people don't have any desire to live into old age is because they are already in poor health. When they think of getting older, they picture themselves in a deteriorated, unhealthy state. C'mon! There are people who are still running marathons in their eighties. You don't have to break down! Expect more from yourself!

Note: If you have a history where all the people in your family die young, it is even more important for you to do this exercise. Do not get caught in the trap of thinking that genetics won't allow you to live a long vital life. We'll talk more about genetics later, but for the time being, just start planning on living a long healthy life.

I plan on living until the age of _____.

Forget Your Diagnosis!

In my practice I've noticed a disturbing trend develop over the last several years. As I discussed in the last chapter, the number of people coming in with chronic health problems and autoimmune conditions is skyrocketing. It seems like a good majority of Americans have some kind of chronic condition or autoimmunity these days. More likely than not, this is due to so much toxicity in present-day life, the amount of stress that people are under, and eating the standard American diet (SAD). If you are one of those people, get ready, because we will discuss real solutions to those problems throughout this book.

If you are not suffering from a chronic health problem or diagnosis, I want you to consider the limitations and/or negative beliefs you have about your physical health as we go through this section of the book.

Unfortunately, many people who are diagnosed with these kinds of problems get a label attached to them, and sometimes they wear that label like a badge of honor. The badge is perpetuated, worsened, and confirmed for these patients with each passing visit to their doctors. They frequently hear comments from their physicians to the effect of, "Well, Mrs. Smith, you have MS. This is just something you will have to learn to live with." Or, "You have fibromyalgia, Ms. Jones. You can expect pain to be part of your everyday life." If I can be frank with you, that attitude totally infuriates me! Before long, these poor people pretty much believe that there is no hope for them, and they begin to own the label. This is why they begin telling their "story," as I discussed in the first chapter.

Owning the label means that they begin to identify themselves with that condition. The labels "fibromyalgia" or "MS" or "Hashimoto's" become interchangeable and synonymous with the person. "My fibromyalgia is acting up today." "My MS is really bothering me today." "My Hashimoto's has really got me tired today." These are common phrases that I hear frequently in my office. When I hear the "my" at the beginning of these sentences, I know that the person in front of me has owned that condition; they believe that there is little hope for them to ever get well. If this is you, *stop it*!

If you suffer from a chronic health problem and you are guilty of owning the label, know that you are not alone and that I know how you feel. When I found out that the reason I had been sick for three years was black mold poisoning, I went through a similar stage. My recovery took a couple of years once we discovered what the problem was, and there were many days when I felt badly and would say things like, "This mold is making me feel tired today." Admittedly, a lot of it was self-pity. But eventually I shook myself free of that label and had to stop saying such things. I knew that if I continued down that road of owning my diagnosis, my chances of recovery would be very slim.

If you want to get past a chronic health problem, if you want to get your life back, you must dissociate yourself from the diagnosis. I'm not suggesting that you pretend you don't have the problem or that you stop any necessary treatments. What I'm saying is that you have to stop thinking your world revolves around condition XYZ. If you want to return to health, you will have to break the habit of identifying yourself with your sickness.

I know you may be thinking, "You're crazy, Dr. Kuhn. I have no desire to identify with my sickness!" I'm not trying to offend anyone, but I'm saying things that I know nobody else will to try and help you. I realize that not all people who suffer from such conditions own their diagnosis or identify themselves with their sickness. But I know from experience that a lot of people do, and if they continue to do so, they will never get well.

For a lot of people, there is tremendous payoff in identifying themselves with their diagnosis. Family members of such patients seem to coddle them, show them regular sympathy, and even relieve them of numerous household duties. I can't tell you how many chronic-condition patients over the years have told me stories about how wonderful their spouse is because he/she does all the laundry, dishes, housework, etc. because they are in too much pain or don't have enough energy to do it. Some people really are too incapacitated to perform such duties, and in those cases I believe it very noble for family members to step in and help. However, not everyone who has been diagnosed with a health problem is incapacitated, and being coddled only enables those people to slide further down the road of futility.

Also, many patients with autoimmunity and chro[...] disability benefits from the government. I'm not [...] those patients don't need that, but I have seen many [...] my office who absolutely should not be on disability. [...] milking the system because of their diagnosis. This is t[...] don't advertise for disability patients, nor do I do disability [...] office. In fact, when patients come into my office who ar[...] ...y on disability, I tell them that if I'm ever requested to write a report for their disability that I will be very honest with my findings. I explain to them that if I feel they are able to work, I will write that in my report. As a result, I don't get too many requests for disability reports. Sadly, some people who come in with a chronic health problem and are on disability drop out of care when they see that what we are doing is getting them better, because they don't want to lose their disability.

To conclude this portion of the chapter, I want you to consider the following things. If what I teach you in this book could completely change your life, would you want it to? Would you be willing to give up the payoffs you have in your life from being chronically ill? If you could get off disability and go back to work, would you do it? If you could again have the energy to run your own life and do your own household chores, would you? Would you be willing to give up all the sympathy and special treatment you receive? This might be tough to think about, I know, but the whole point I want you to get out of this is that you must be willing to leave your diagnosis behind and stop believing that you are your condition. You are not, and your life can be so much more.

Creating the New You

I am now going to walk you through a drill where we will create the vision of a beautiful, healthy, new you. My hope is that you will give this your best effort because it will be a springboard to your success as we go through the rest of the book.

Please read all the way through this drill before you begin so you get a complete understanding of what it is I am asking you to do. Once you have read through the whole explanation, spend about twenty minutes visualizing everything that I have described in the recommend that you do this visualization technique every day for twenty-one days. I want you to develop a strong habit of perceiving yourself as your best, healthiest self.

Don't haphazardly try to rush through this drill. Find a nice, quiet place where you won't be disturbed. I recommend a favorite comfortable chair, yoga mat, or other relaxing place that you favor. Give yourself at least twenty minutes to complete this drill without interruptions. Turn off your cell phone and make sure nothing else like barking dogs or electronic equipment might disturb you. Let's get started.

We are going to do a visualization technique. In order for this to be effective, it is very important that you do your best to actually feel the sensations and visuals that are being described. In other words, don't just see them—feel them.

I want you to close your eyes and picture yourself walking along a beach, in the mountains or a country meadow. Choose a setting that is very pleasing to you. Picture yourself in a swimsuit or gym clothing so you can get a full view of your body. As you are walking along the beach, feel the cool ocean breeze or mountain air upon your face as you notice the clean smell of nature. Take in some deep healing breaths, and feel a tremendous sense of calm about you. Pause right now, breathe deeply, and notice this feeling. There is nothing to stress about, no problems to be concerned with. Notice that you feel very grateful for your body and that you feel fabulous in it. Repeat these words in your head, or out loud if you feel comfortable: I am so grateful for my healthy body.

Now, picture what your body looks and feels like from the ground up. As you observe your legs, notice that they are leaner, stronger, and functioning perfectly. There is no pain or improper joint motion in your feet, ankles, knees, or hips. Happily notice that they seem to be moving and feeling better than they ever have. Delighted by this, you decide to test your new lower body by going for a short jog. You are astonished to discover that you just easily jogged a few hundred yards without exertion, pain, or discomfort.

Moving upwards, you notice that your derrière, waistline, and abdomen are in better shape than you ever thought possible. Imagine what that would look like to you. Furthermore, you notice that your whole gastrointestinal system feels very comfortable. You seem to have perfect digestion, and there is nothing but calm in your belly. It's a great feeling.

The first thing you notice about your chest is that your heart is beating in a perfect, slow, restful, rhythm, and it feels strong, really strong. Your breaths are easy, your lungs feel strong and the thought crosses your mind that you could truly do anything you wanted to right now. Physically, your chest looks the way you've always wanted it to. Whether you are male or female, imagine what that looks like to you. The most astounding thing though is that your energy level seems to be different. In fact, you are experiencing more energy in your body than you have since childhood. You are thinking clearly, seeing clearly, and you feel very much in touch with your surroundings. You think that you could run forever.

Your shoulders move and function perfectly. They have excellent range of motion, and you are very pleased to see that the tone and shape of your arms is wonderful. All of your upper body joints move well and feel great.

Aesthetically, your skin is glowing and looks clear and healthy. Your appearance makes you feel ecstatic about yourself. Once again, let out a deep, slow breath, grateful that you are alive in this fantastic body.

Your spine and back feel very flexible. Amazingly, your back is loose, and you feel taller and more upright than you ever have. There are no aches and pains. In awe of this, you stop walking and decide to test out your back and hips. You easily bend down and touch your toes and effortlessly move your torso from side to side and rotate back and forth. *Incredible!* you think. You feel absolutely incredible.

In love with your healthy new body, you sit down on the beach facing the ocean, or in a perfect spot on a beautiful mountain just in time to watch the sun set. A beautiful breeze wisps through your hair, and again you appreciate the smell of nature. Feeling phenomenal, you slowly breathe in and out, thanking your body for how good you feel. Before finishing this visualization, relax into this setting for a few moments, and feel the serenity.

What Next?

First of all, it is important when doing this drill not to get caught up in semantics. If you don't like the way I described something, change it to something that makes you feel comfortable. There is one thing you absolutely cannot change, though: no matter how you walk yourself through this drill, you must make it so that all your body systems function and feel perfect! Even if you have a prosthetic leg, a pacemaker, or some other disability, visualize yourself as perfectly healthy. I want you to develop no-limit thinking!

I still do this drill on a regular basis, and it always keeps me focused on what I need to do. If you are in dire need of a health overhaul, I recommend you do this drill once a day, every day, for three months. Another great way to do this visualization is to do it while you go for a walk in the early morning hours. If you choose this, leave the IPod at home and simply visualize and listen to the sounds of nature.

From this day forward, I want you to truly believe that you are healthy. When you are faced with a health challenge, I want you to realize that you can overcome it and to commit to doing whatever necessary to make it so. You have your whole life in front of you, and you need to think of it that way, regardless of what age you currently are. Remember, fifty is the new thirty. If you are eighty years old right now, you could still have quite a number of years left, so why not live them to the fullest? It's truly time to start living!

Action Steps

- Define what good health means to you. Write in your journal a definition of what having good health means to you

- Plan your own death: Decide what age you want to live to. Write it down

- Dissociate yourself from any diagnosis or condition—stop believing that your condition runs your life

- Decide that you will give up whatever payoffs you may be getting from your condition

- Do the "Creating the New You" drill with feeling and purpose

Chapter 5

Detoxification

As the body begins to make gains via detoxification, it
then turns its attention to breaking down and removing
diseased cells, replacing them with healthy ones.

—Ron Garner

If you were born and raised in the United States, there is more
than a good chance that by the time you were six months old you
already had numerous highly toxic chemicals injected into your body
via childhood immunizations. Regardless of what your stance is on
vaccinations, do not for one second believe that they don't contain
many harmful toxic elements. They do. That's a fact. It is astounding
to me that specific hazardous material disposal methods have to be
utilized to dispose of them, but they are deemed safe to inject into
the human body.

The chemical soup that was deliberately put into your body as a child is vast. A plethora of antibiotics, cough syrups, and fever-reducing medications were probably put into your body by the time you were two years old.

The purpose of this chapter is not to stir up a debate or persuade you not to vaccinate. The point I wanted to make with the opening paragraphs is that your body has already been in a state of high toxicity almost since the day you were born, and it's wrecking your health. To truly discover a life of optimal health and improve your chances for longer life, getting rid of the toxins in your body is an absolute requirement. If you have any type of chronic health problem or autoimmune condition, the importance of detoxification cannot be overlooked.

Why Detox?

Detoxification, or "detoxing," is very common in natural healthcare circles these days. Those of us who try to be on the cutting edge have known about the incredible powers of detox for quite some time.

I must say that I am sometimes surprised by some doctors' tendencies to dismiss the necessity for detoxing, which to me is just common sense. Let me give you a simple analogy. Suppose the water in your swimming pool was nasty looking because your filters were clogged up with leaves, dirt, and other debris. It wouldn't make sense to try and improve the water by adding chlorine without cleaning out the filters, would it? Of course not. By adding chlorine without cleaning out the filters, at best you might see better-looking water for a couple of days before it started turning murky again.

Likewise, it doesn't make much sense to start eating healthier, exercising and taking supplements in an attempt to improve your health if your body's tissues and organs are still clogged up with a plethora of toxins. Those toxins create a cesspool. They are sickness, disease, and poor health just waiting to happen.

Lastly, your body truly is your temple. I am a firm believer that we are spiritual beings having a physical experience, to borrow a popular phrase. That being said, I really believe that having a body that is mucked-up and congested with toxicity is a sure way to block access to your soul. If you doubt that statement, ask yourself if you think a cocaine addict or an alcoholic has clear access to his or her soul. The simple act of reaching again and again in an addictive manner for something like cocaine or alcohol is an indication that a person is cut off from his or her soul. I'm not suggesting that you can't be a spiritual person or have spiritual beliefs if you have addiction problems, but you are certainly not living from your spirit. If you were, you would not need the substance you are addicted to. To live an inspired life, you must be in tune, spiritually, mentally, and physically.

> # What is the point of being alive if you don't at least try to do something remarkable?

Detox What?

So what exactly should you be interested in detoxing? Your fingernails? Your shoes? It would probably be helpful to know exactly what parts of the body would most benefit from a detox and how that would affect your physiology. But I'd like to go one step further and suggest that you should really consider detoxing your life, not just your body.

With all the research on detoxification that has been done in the last several years showing how different nutritional compounds can target specific organs, you can literally detox just about any part of the body you want. For example, we carry a full-body detox in my office that detoxes the digestive system, liver, gallbladder, lungs, kidneys, bladder, lymphatic system, blood, and skin. However, it isn't necessary for most people to do that much detoxing. In fact, the majority of people who decide to purchase that particular detox are very healthy and proactive in taking care of themselves. But what about the average person? What about you? What kind of detox should you do?

By the time most Americans have reached the age of twenty, they are in serious need of cleaning out their gastrointestinal system (which we will call the gut) and their liver. This probably includes you. By the time we are in our thirties, our guts and livers are toxic enough to start an avalanche of bad health. For this reason, the gut and liver is where I recommend starting with detoxing.

Think about it. The job of these two organs is to filter out all the junk that goes through your body, much like your pool filter cleans out leaves, dirt, and debris in your swimming pool. The gut and liver have a hard enough job doing what they do in people who take good care of themselves; the majority of people in our country treat their bodies like a garbage dump. Your gut and liver are largely responsible for maintaining an optimal level of health in your body. In fact, it is estimated that 80 percent of all disease starts in the gut; I agree with that statement. As I stated earlier, it's challenging enough for the gut and liver to do their jobs in healthy people. Imagine how difficult and compromising it is for those organs to do their jobs properly in people who are living shoddy lifestyles. Is it any wonder that so many people are suffering from chronically poor health in our country? Not remotely!

Unfortunately, in traditional Western medicine, the gut is rarely paid any attention as a source of chronic health problems. Unless you go into your doctor's office complaining of acid reflux–like symptoms or you bleed when you have a bowel movement, your gut will not be given much credence. But because of how the gut works and what takes place there, in cases of chronically bad health it should be the first system to address. Let me repeat that: in chronically bad health, the gut should be the first system to address. To illustrate this point, the following is a very short list of important processes that occur in the gut.

- Some conversion of thyroid hormones (the rest takes place in the liver)

- Salivary IgA: this is the first line of immune system defense in the body

- Processing of vitamin B-12

- Absorption of vitamins and minerals from food

- Maintaining a balanced environment of bacteria

I listed only five processes here to illustrate a point. Due to toxicity or toxicity-related conditions, each of these activities can be affected. Compromising these five activities could account for problems related to the following:

- Hypothyroidism

- Chronic sicknesses (recurring colds, allergies, etc.)

- Chronic fatigue

- Chronic pain syndromes (fibromyalgia)

- Lack of energy

- Irritable bowel syndrome

- Crohn's disease

- Ulcerative colitis

- Adrenal stress syndrome

- Depression

- Megaloblastic anemia

- Food sensitivities

- Neurodegeneration

- Cardiovascular disease

- Inability to lose weight

As you can see, just a few seemingly innocuous things being out of balance can lead to a whole litany of health problems.

A Stunning Story of Bad Gut Health!

Recently, a fifty-one-year-old female came to see me with global body pain that had been diagnosed as fibromyalgia. We'll call her Jane. After consulting with her and doing an initial physical exam, she told me that she had also been suffering with ulcerative colitis. If you are not familiar with ulcerative colitis, it is an autoimmune condition where the sufferer has lesions in the gut that produce frequent or constant bleeding, inflammation, nodules, and polyps. Basically, every time someone with ulcerative colitis goes to the bathroom, the result is a toilet full of blood. You can imagine how uncomfortable that is.

In the medical model, these patients are typically put on powerful sulfur drugs and sometimes steroids to manage the condition. If the condition gets bad enough, it can lead to colon cancer, so many of these patients end up having part of their colon removed and have to use a colostomy bag to empty their feces for the rest of their lives. Obviously, that is a bad situation.

That Jane had colitis was crucial information for me to learn, because gut conditions like that can lead to chronic pain syndromes like fibromyalgia. I might be providing someone with the best chiropractic treatment in the world, but if a patient has an inflamed gut, their pain levels may not decrease. I immediately asked Jane to do a five-day food diary for me. I asked her to write down everything she ate, drank, or put in her mouth for five days. When Jane brought the food diary back to me I was astonished at what I saw. Her food diary was dominated by such foods as french fries, pizza, ice cream, licorice, garlic bread, peanut butter sandwiches, potato chips, pop tarts, hash browns, diet Cokes, popcorn, and chocolate cake. Other than some bananas, I was hard pressed to find anything of nutritional value on the list. But one thing really intrigued me. I noticed that on each day she wrote down "six gumballs." I asked her about it, and she said, "You know, the old-fashioned gumballs." But what she said next was the real eye-opener. She said, "You don't know the worst part, Dr. Rob."

"What's that?" I asked.

She replied, "I eat them."

So I asked her how long she had been eating gumballs. She responded that she had been doing that for years. I was blown away to say the least.

I was excited at the information I had learned from doing her food diary and confident that we could help her make some very positive changes. I quickly started Jane on a liver and gut detox, which included a modified diet and supplementation. Within just a couple of weeks, she was no longer bleeding from her colon, her body aches had diminished to almost none, and she lost over thirty pounds to boot! A miracle, right? Well, it would be if it were an isolated incident. The reality is that in functional medicine, we see results such as these frequently.

Shortly after we began to see improvement, Jane commented that her gastroenterologist had never once even asked her about her diet. Think about that. The doctor who is a "specialist" in treating the organ that is responsible for digesting and processing food had never once asked her about diet! Don't you think that's a pretty important factor for someone who has a bleeding colon? Me too.

What About the Rest of Your Life?

I've already talked about why you should detox. I'm going to offer some "how-to" in a moment, but first I'd like to talk about what other things in your life could be causing toxicity in your body.

It is very challenging for me to put detox into one chapter. I could write an entire book on this topic alone. There is so much to it; so many different things fit into the "detox envelope." But my goal is to keep it simple and to give you basic working knowledge that will allow you to immediately see positive changes in your life.

Toxicity is all around you, and it is affecting you and your loved ones, whether you realize it or not. Unless you have already gone "green," chances are that toxic chemicals are in all of your household cleaning supplies, your carpets, the clothes on your back, your food, your toothpaste, and your personal hygiene products. These few areas are a very short list, but it is a great place for us to start.

Let me start by covering a few of the ones you can make immediate changes to.

Household cleaning supplies: Most of these products contain harmful ingredients like:

- ammonias, which can cause pulmonary and cardiovascular problems

- glycol ethers, which can lead to blood disorders, liver problems, and kidney damage

- phenols, which are known as gender benders for causing hormonal shift problems

Food: If you aren't a conscious shopper, your food most likely contains numerous pesticides, herbicides, fungicides, and carcinogens.

Personal hygiene products: Below is a short list of the almost 85,000 different toxic chemicals that are used in making personal products. Almost all personal hygiene products contain some ingredients like:

- stearic acid: potential carcinogen

- sorbitol: potential carcinogen

71

- glycerin: potential carcinogen

- alkyl benzoate: potential carcinogen

- sodium borate: potential carcinogen

- methyl paraben: potential carcinogen

- propylene glycol: potential carcinogen

- cetyl alcohol: potential carcinogen

- aluminum: linked to Alzheimer's disease

- fluoride: highly toxic, no matter what your dentist says

Hopefully, you are starting to get the picture of how toxic your life probably is. I know that most people's response when learning of these issues is to think that if these chemicals were really that toxic to the body, the FDA would never allow their use. Many patients in my workshops make that very statement. As discussed in chapter 2, you will be much better off if you just realize and accept that the FDA is not looking out for your best interests. If you are still unsure, I challenge you to do your own research. Google these chemicals and see what you find.

Bottom line: if you want to live a long, healthy, pain-free life, you must start detoxifying your personal environment.

How Toxic Is Your Life?

Before you give yourself an out, I want to reiterate that what most people consider living a healthy lifestyle is not even in the same stratosphere as what I would consider living a healthy lifestyle. In fact, I am sometimes very surprised by what people consider to be a healthy lifestyle. If you would like to find out how healthy your lifestyle really is, I challenge you to take the following quiz. At the end, we will rate where you stand on my scale of a healthy lifestyle.

For each question, mark the answer that best describes your life. Be sure to answer each question as honestly as you can. Remember, this is for your eyes only. The outcome you will get from this will be invaluable.

1. I stop at fast food restaurants such as McDonald's, Wendy's, Burger King, Taco Bell, Jack in the Box, Chick Fil A, Hardees, Whataburger, KFC, etc. …

   A. Never
   B. Once per month
   C. Once per week
   D. Two times per week or more

2. I smoke cigarettes …

   A. Never
   B. Only when I drink alcohol
   C. At least 5 cigarettes per day
   D. More than 5 cigarettes per day

3. I use marijuana or other recreational drugs …

   A. Never
   B. Occasionally at parties or social events
   C. At least one time per month
   D. At least one time per week

4. My consumption of alcohol is …

   A. Never
   B. 1–2 drinks per week
   C. 3–7 drinks per week
   D. 8 or more drinks per week

5. I drink soda or diet soda …

   A. Never   C. 1 soda per day
   B. 1–3 sodas per   D. 2 or more sodas per day
      week

6. I eat potato chips, pretzels, Pringles, etc …

   A. Never   C. 2–3 times per week
   B. 1 time per week   D. more than 3 times per
                                  week

7. I eat processed food from a box or a bag such as cereal, rice, Hamburger Helper, etc. …

   A. Never   C. 2–3 times per week
   B. About once per   D. More than 3 times per
      week   week

8. I do a *planned exercise routine* at least … (walking around at your job or some other type of random walking does not count)

   A. 5–7 days per week   C. 1–2 days per week
   B. 3–4 days per week   D. Never

9. I take over-the-counter medications including but not limited to: NSAIDS like Tylenol, Advil, aspirin, etc., sinus meds like Allegra, Afrin, etc., cold and flu meds like Nyquil, etc., Pepto Bismol, or any other over-the-counter drugs …

   A. In extreme cases,   C. 1-2 times per week
      maybe 1-2 times
      per year.
   B. 1–2 times per   D. Daily
      month

10. I take prescription medication …

    A. Only in extreme cases, maybe once every couple of years.

    B. Roughly a few times per year

    C. Several times per year.

    D. On a regular basis

11. The following statement best represents my sleeping habits:

    A. I go to bed and wake up at the same time every day

    B. I go to bed at the same time every night, but wake up at a different time each day.

    C. I go to bed at a different time every night, but wake up at the same time each day

    D. I go to bed at a different time every night and wake up at a different time every day.

12. I get at least …

    A. 7–8 hours of sleep/night

    B. 6–7 hours of sleep/night

    C. 5–6 hours of sleep/ night

    D. less than 5 hours of sleep/night

13. I take natural vitamin supplements such as multivitamins, vitamin C, Vitamin D or other common vitamins …

    A. On a consistent daily basis

    B. A couple of times per week

    C. Whenever I remember to take them

    D. Never

14. I eat a good healthy salad (not a huge restaurant salad that is loaded with junk) …

    A. 5–7 times per week

    B. 3–4 times per week

    C. 1–2 times per week

    D. Maybe once or twice per month or less

15. I would rate my stress level as follows:

    A. Low stress

    B. Moderate stress

    C. High stress

    D. Off the charts

16. I would best describe my feelings toward my job as: (If you are a homemaker, that is a full-time job, so do answer this question.)

    A. I love my job

    B. My job is okay

    C. I don't like my job

    D. I hate my job

17. My consumption of pure, clean, filtered water is closest to …

    A. 4 or more glasses per day

    B. 3 glasses per day

    C. 2 glasses per day

    D. 1 glass per day or less

18. In regards to television, I watch … (this includes DVDs, sports, TiVo, etc.)

    A. 1 hour or less per day

    B. 2 hours or less per day

    C. 3 hours per day

    D. 4 or more hours per day

19. I eat candy, desserts, donuts, or other sweets ...

    A. Maybe 1–2 times   C. Once per day
       per week

    B. Several times per   D. More than once per day
       week

20. When shopping for beef, chicken, fish, or vegetables, I specifically look for organic, all-natural, top quality products ...

    A. Always   C. If I happen to think
                            about it

    B. Sometimes   D. Never; it is too expensive, and they aren't any different anyways.

21. I eat different kinds of bread, restaurant bread, biscuits, or muffins ... (Include all of your meals)

    A. A couple of pieces   C. 3–4 pieces/day or less
       per week or less

    B. 1–2 pieces/day or   D. more than 4 pieces per
       less   day

22. I eat pasta, noodles, or rice ...

    A. once a week or less   C. 4–6 times a week
    B. 2–3 times a week   D. every day

23. I use either Equal or Splenda as a sugar substitute ...

    A. Never   C. On a semi-regular basis
    B. Occasionally   D. Every day

24. I sit in front of a computer for approximately …

    A. Less than one
       hour per day

    B. 1–2 hours per day

    C. 3–4 hours per day

    D. More than 5 hours per
       day

25. In regards to my personal hygiene products and household cleaning supplies:

    A. I buy all organic

    B. I try to buy
       natural products

    C. I buy the most popular
       brands

    D. I buy the cheapest stuff
       I can find

Now it's time to tally up your score. Go through and assign the following point value to each corresponding letter that you answered.

A — 1 point

B — 2 points

C — 3 points

D — 4 points

Once you have assigned your point values, add up the total of all of your points.

The lowest possible score you can have on this quiz is 25; the highest is 100. If you scored exactly 25, count yourself among the healthiest people on the planet. If you scored exactly 100, I hope you have your life insurance and your last will and testament updated, because they will be put to use sooner rather than later. I'm not joking.

(25–35) If you scored in this category, congratulations—you are living a healthy lifestyle. You probably have a serious plan for your health and how you take care of your body. There is a good chance that you have goals for your future and you have a bright outlook on life. Most likely, you rarely experience health problems, and if you do, you are probably quick to heal. Look for ideas in this book for how you can improve, and keep up the good work.

(36–49) This category can be tricky. If you are in this group you may be someone who does pay some attention to your health, or you may just have landed here by accident. It's possible that you may have been raised by parents who had some natural wisdom to teach about how to take care of yourself, or you may have started to educate yourself about healthy living. Only you can know which of those scenarios is true for you. If you are in this group, you are doing okay, but make no mistake—you want to try and move into the first category. Go back through your quiz and note the questions that you answered with either C or D. Ask yourself how you can upgrade those answers to an A or B. While your lifestyle is already fairly good, don't get cocky. It can go south in a hurry. Look for clues in this book about how you can keep improving.

(50—74) If your score is over 50, I have six words for you: wake up before it's too late! You are on a collision course toward bad health. You are likely someone who gets sick a few times per year; you might deal with several bouts of random aches and pains as well. There is a good chance that you feel older than you are. In fact, you might be someone who frequently justifies your feelings of lost vigor and vitality with the phrase, "I'm just getting older." You quickly need to make lifestyle changes to avoid becoming someone who has chronic pain and autoimmune deficiencies. At this point, you can either make a turn toward health or you can continue to slide into the abyss. Which will you choose?

(75–100) You are a toxic train wreck! Earlier I said that if you scored 100 you'd better make sure your life insurance and last will and testament are updated because you'll be needing them sooner rather later. If your score is over 75, the same applies, so I'm glad you got to read that sentence twice. As I'm sure you're probably aware from your atrocious health, these are desperate times for you, and they call for desperate measures. More likely than not you get sick frequently or you have constant symptoms of discomfort or lowered health in your body. The medicine cabinet at your house is probably stocked full of over-the-counter pain medications, drugs for upset stomachs, sinus and allergy relievers, and sleeping pills. You probably couldn't tell me the last time you ate a salad. The other people living in your house are likely as sick as you are. Many people in your shoes are well aware that their lifestyle is destroying their health, though many have no idea. This is a defining moment for you. If you don't make the decision to change your life right now, it soon may be too late.

The good news is that no matter where you fall on this grading scale, there is room for improvement. You can change your life! Yes, even you toxic train wrecks can make a complete turnaround. I have seen people whose health could best be characterized as absolute disasters make a 180-degree turn and end up living an amazingly healthy and inspired life. You can too! You must believe that. It's not your job to doubt. It's your job to make the decision to get healthier. For the time being, just trust me. Put one foot in front of the other, and let's get you moving toward good health.

The Three Areas to Detox

As I see it, just about every aspect of your life that needs to be detoxed can be broken down into three main components: physical, mental, and spiritual. In the interest of keeping brief, I'm only going to focus on the physical aspect of detox here. However, I will say that the mental and spiritual aspects can create just as much discomfort, pain, and sickness in your life as the physical. I will talk about mental and spiritual health in the last chapter, but all of the toxic stuff that you are carrying around resides in one of these three areas. Let's examine the physical and see what actions you can take to start living a less toxic life.

Physical

As I discussed in the beginning of this chapter, with existing products, you could literally detoxify just about any part of the body that you want. However, I want to keep it simple. As far as your organs go, let's stick to the gut and liver. If you have chronic pain, autoimmune problems, or any undesired state of health, it is crucial to take care of these. I feel so strongly about this that I always do a liver and gut detox every year. It's that important.

The gut: Aside from all the junk that accumulates in the gut, we want to work on solving problems like dysbiosis, leaky gut syndrome, hypochlorhydria, and parasite infections. Below is a brief definition of each of these conditions in lay terms.

Dysbiosis: a condition where there is an imbalance between the good and bad bacteria in your gut

Leaky gut syndrome: a condition where the intestinal tract lining becomes damaged, allowing toxins, and certain particles of undigested waste to pass through the gut wall. This can result in discomfort, inflammation, pain, and autoimmune flare-ups, but it can also be present without symptoms.

Hypochlorhydria: a condition where insufficient stomach acid is produced. This will cause food to *not* be properly digested, allowing food to become putrid in your stomach. The result will be symptoms that mimic acid reflux, although the problem is actually a shortage of stomach acid, whereas acid reflux is thought to be caused by too much stomach acid.

Parasites: bugs get into your gut and may cause numerous health problems. The majority of these will go undetected by traditional medical testing.

The liver: Because the liver is a filtering system, it too will accumulate a lot of junk, which necessitates detoxing. In the liver we want to solve problems like sluggish liver and fatty liver.

Sluggish liver: your liver is just tired and toxic. We call this having a sluggish liver. The liver is clogged up and having a hard time doing its job.

Fatty liver: too much fat is stored in the cells of the liver. Fatty liver is very common in cases of regular alcohol usage and chronically bad diets.

Detoxing the gut and liver

To properly detox the gut and liver, a very specific diet protocol and supplementation program must be followed. Because so many possible health conditions can be associated with these organs, this is the only part of the book where I will not just tell you how to do it by using store bought supplements and trying it by yourself.

First of all, I don't use store-bought supplements, as most of them are of questionable quality. Secondly, I believe that for a liver-gut detox, you should be under the care of a doctor with specific training in nutrition and functional medicine.

In other chapters in the book I will give you specific, easy-to-follow steps to make immediate improvements in your health. But I believe it is of the utmost importance that this detox be done correctly and under a doctor's supervision. If you are currently under the care of a chiropractor, an acupuncturist, or a naturopathic doctor, ask them about doing a detox related to the conditions I listed above. If you don't feel confident that they are familiar with it, or you would like to consult with me about this, visit my website to schedule a consultation.

One thing that will mildly detox your liver and improve your overall health is drinking water with lemon every day. Lemon provides a mild detox for the body that will be helpful to you.

Heavy Metals

It may be necessary for you to do some kind of chelation therapy to detox heavy metals out of your body. Many people can have elevated levels of mercury or other heavy metals, which can make it difficult or impossible for you to ever achieve optimal health. In my office, we utilize hair analysis testing to determine heavy metal toxicity.

Heavy metals can in fact be the source of chronic health problems for some people. In some cases, those "mysterious" undiagnosed conditions can be the result of heavy metal toxicity.

Although I only wrote a short section about this type of toxicity, it can be one of the more significant areas to address, so don't underestimate it's importance. It is critically important to note that you should not do any chelation therapy if you still have mercury amalgam fillings in your teeth. This will move mercury around different parts of your brain and body and you don't want that. Of equal importance is finding a dentist that uses I.A.O.M.T. protocols for mercury amalgam removal. If you have a natural healthcare practitioner you are happy with, ask them about detoxing for heavy metals. If not, contact me and we will see about getting you set up.

Food: I will be covering food issues in detail in the next chapter. For now, let me just leave you with this thought: *stop eating so much crap*! It's as simple as that. The food choices that you make are largely responsible for the majority of toxicity in your body, which is why in the next chapter I am going to teach you once and for all how to eat.

Household Products: Regarding your household products and personal hygiene products—you must make the switch to organic now! It is time. You must start using all-natural organic products. The majority of grocery stores now have an organic section filled with all-natural products, from household cleaners to laundry detergents and personal hygiene products.

Hygiene Products: As far as hygiene, I consider the two most important items to discuss to be deodorants and toothpastes. The majority of deodorants on the market are loaded with aluminum. Aluminum is a toxic element that you don't want in your body. It has been linked to Alzheimer's disease, and elevated levels will lead to neurological degeneration. You can find a plethora of natural deodorants in most grocery stores.

As for toothpaste, fluoride is a major cause of toxicity. If you want to learn more about fluoride toxicity, go to www.mercola.com and search fluoride. You will find more reading on this issue than you'll ever have time for. You can find natural toothpastes in your grocery store.

Personal Environment: Be sure that you are not living in a home, apartment, etc., that is infested with mold, rot, or other toxic problems. After my mold experience, I am shocked at how many people I have since met who are knowingly living in a home with mold in it. Some of them have told me that their doctors have said it's not that big a deal. Let me tell you, it is a huge deal! It can make you deathly ill or even kill you. If you know you have mold in your house, do not attempt to clean it with bleach or anything else, as that will only spread it and make it worse. You need to either have a professional mold remediation or move out. If I knew then what I know now, I would have left my house the day we found out about the mold and never looked back.

Cigarettes: Really? Do I even need to write about this? It's 2012. The research has been done. It astonishes me that with all the knowledge that is out there that anybody on planet Earth still smokes cigarettes. I watched my mother die a horrible, painful death from smoking-related illnesses at the age of sixty-three. Some patients who come into my office are smokers, and I can't help but think as I look at them that the end of their life will come sooner than expected, and it won't be a peaceful ending. It has been my experience that large portions of fibromyalgia patients are smokers. Sadly, because their cells are being deprived of oxygen, these patients have a long shot at ever regaining a healthy, happy life. If you smoke, just stop, and stop now. No excuses, no waiting—just do it. It will be the best decision you've ever made.

Alcohol: I am not completely opposed to alcohol. I enjoy a glass of wine or a cocktail as much as the next person. The problem is when alcohol becomes an everyday outlet for your problems and/or becomes abused. Make no mistake; too much alcohol is very toxic to the body. If you drink daily, cut back to every other day and then to just a couple of drinks per week. If you have a problem, get help. Remember, a healthy liver is a big key to a long, happy life. Use common sense.

Just the Tip of the Iceberg

When it comes to detoxing, I have just scraped the tip of the iceberg in this chapter. In our country, we have an alarming problem with the rise of cancers, autoimmune problems, chronic pain syndromes, and overall poor health. Much of this is due to the toxic choices we make every day. If you want to regain your health and live an incredibly passionate, energetic life, you must become less toxic.

Important Note: As discussed earlier, if you suffer from a chronic health problem, or any autoimmune problem, it is *critical* that you detox your gut and liver. Liver and gut problems are not necessarily the cause, but are involved with most chronic health problems. It may not make sense to you that having a bad gut or a toxic liver could be related to fibromyalgia, Sjogren's syndrome, hypothyroidism, or any other chronic health problem, but they are. The systemic inflammation that results from these problems can cause mayhem all over the body. I cannot even begin to stress how important it is to have these systems function properly. If these systems have not been approached properly, your chances of a full recovery are very slim. Be sure to take action on this with a qualified natural healthcare professional.

Action Steps

- Review your toxic lifestyle evaluation and highlight all the areas that you marked C or D. Find ways to move these answers into the A or B level.

- Begin utilizing all-natural household cleaning supplies.

- Make the switch to all-natural organic personal hygiene products.

- Become a conscious shopper and seek out the best in all-natural organic foods.

- Consult with a natural healthcare practitioner or visit my website and get started on a liver-gut detox immediately.

- If you are a smoker, decide what methods you will use to quit and get started.

- If you consume alcohol, begin to cut back on the amount of your consumption.

Chapter 6

Do You Know How To Eat?

Let thy food be thy medicine, and thy medicine be thy food.

—Hippocrates

In my second year of practice, a male patient in his late thirties approached me about weight loss. He weighed over four hundred pounds and was seriously considering having gastric bypass surgery. I was elated that he came to me first because I was very familiar with the awful statistics and outcomes of gastric bypass surgery.

As fate would have it, within just a few days of my meeting with that patient, several others inquired about weight loss too. Confident that I could do better than what was out there, I decided to hold my first weight-loss seminar for my patient base so I could teach them all at the same time.

We had thirty-nine people show up for that first seminar. I taught them my version of weight loss and put them all on a twelve-week plan. At our twelve-week goal date, the four hundred–pound patient had lost over ninety pounds! A few others lost around sixty pounds, and several others lost between twenty and forty pounds. Not bad for the first time. That experience lit a fire in me that drives a strong passion to help people with weight loss. I have held an annual weight-loss seminar every year since then for my patient base. Typically anywhere between fifty and one hundred people show up. Of all the talks I do in my practice, this topic has the greatest attendance by far. Clearly, the general public is in dire need of solid advice on how to eat.

This Is the One

Despite the fact that I opened this chapter with a story about weight loss, what I will present here goes way beyond that. While I will tell you how to lose weight if you're interested, this chapter is about eating to change your life. When it comes to helping people get well, as a doctor of chiropractic who also practices functional medicine, I have a lot of tricks in my bag. There are numerous paths to take to help a patient regain health. But if you pinned me down and told me I could only use one approach on every patient who came to me for help, without question it would be proper nutrition.

Everything that I discuss in this book is very important to regaining your health and to living a long vibrant life, but make no mistake, *this is the one*! Not one component of your lifestyle is as important to your overall health as learning how to properly fuel your body. It doesn't matter how well you may think you're doing right now—if you want to avoid being a healthcare statistic, you must learn how to eat! Am I making myself clear?

Over the years, many patients have come to me whose health was literally in shambles because of how they had treated their own bodies for the majority of their lives. You must understand that everything you put into your mouth will affect the biochemistry of every single cell in your body. In the last chapter I said you must stop toxifying. Well, if you are eating toxic food every day of your life, which most people are, you are killing yourself ... literally. You are damaging tissues and cells in your body and causing them to malfunction. This is one of the reasons why you can be cruising through life in seemingly good health when all of sudden, from out of nowhere—wham! You suddenly have chest pains, or problems digesting food, or chronic fatigue syndrome, and you rack your brain trying to figure out why this "all of a sudden" happened to you.

There is one concept I really want you to get and it is this: you do not catch disease; you develop disease. You don't catch cancer; you develop cancer. You don't catch diabetes; you develop diabetes. You don't catch chronic fatigue; you develop chronic fatigue. You don't catch bad health; you develop bad health. They are a process. You don't catch them like a cold. They build up over time and then—wham! They hit you over the head, as if they came on suddenly, when in reality they have been developing for a long time.

Take my mold symptoms, for example. Once we discovered why we were sick, the contractors determined that the water leak under our house that caused the mold growth had probably been going on since the day we moved in; the mold had started growing immediately. But I didn't start having mold symptoms the day we moved in. No, it took a few months of repeated exposure to those mold toxins before my body got sick. It didn't happen overnight; it was a process that developed in my body. But when it hit me, believe me, it felt like it had happened overnight.

The point I'm trying to drive home is that how you choose to fuel your body will significantly determine the level of your overall health. If you eat food that is void of actual nutrition, you will at some point in your life develop sickness and/or disease. Garbage in = garbage out! You can count on it. If this becomes your reality, you will be at the mercy of a medical system that will put you on numerous medications to try and manage your poor health. The medications won't work, though, because medications can't fix a bad lifestyle. The medication that you are put on, which is toxic, will then become part of your poor lifestyle and poor health; the problem will snowball, and you will get worse and worse. Unfortunately, tens of millions of Americans are living the nightmare I just described. Unless they wake up and make some changes, there is no hope for them.

On the flip side, if you eat real food that is packed with nutrients, you will more likely than not live a vibrant life with good health, void of sickness or disease. Health in = health out! You can count on that too. If this becomes your reality, you will then be living a life that will make most people say you are lucky. You won't need medicine. You will make more and more good choices for your body, which will improve your health; your energy levels will go up, and you will find yourself doing more of the things you love to do. That is what life is all about!

First and Foremost: Proper pH

One of the first steps in creating optimal health is to make sure your body has a proper pH. Ideally, you want your pH to be more on the alkaline side. The best way to test your body pH is through urinalysis. You would like your pH to be between 6.4 and 7.0.

The way you achieve an alkaline pH is by eating more live foods. This is why juicing and eating raw foods is so beneficial. I would say if you have cancer that you don't even have a choice. I am not a vegetarian, but I do advocate eating at least fifty percent of your diet as raw foods.

You more likely than not need to supplement with a top quality mineral as well. If your pH is below 6.0 that means you are very acidic. Most Americans live in an acidic state. When you are acidic, calcium gets stripped from your bones, which leaves you open to becoming osteoporotic. Your body is also oxygen depleted when you are acidic. Mineral supplementation is crucial.

I know there are numerous companies out there selling "alkaline water." They are also selling home systems to alkalinize your water. I'm sorry to tell you, but drinking alkaline water will not alkalinize your body. I wouldn't waste my money. The key is eating live foods and mineral supplementation.

> The distance between dreams
> and reality is called *discipline*!

How Humans Should Eat

Up until the last couple of hundred years, the incidence of heart disease, cancer, diabetes, chronic fatigue syndrome, ADHD, and a plethora of other common modern maladies were next to nonexistent. As a matter of fact, if you go back to the earliest humans on planet Earth, they more likely than not didn't have any of that stuff. Of course they had to worry about being eaten by saber-tooth tigers, being killed by other members of an unruly civilization, or dying of the plague. But I'm pretty sure they weren't concerned about blood sugar issues, migraine headaches, or high cholesterol.

As a general rule, you always want your food to be as close to its God-created form as possible. In other words, your food should be as close as possible to the natural form that it arrived on planet Earth. Think frozen vegetables versus fresh vegetables. If you had a bushel of fresh, organic broccoli and a box of frozen broccoli sitting on a table next to each other, you could clearly see that the fresh bushel is in its natural form; the frozen version was processed to fit into a box for storage and freezing. You see the difference, right? I'm telling you, healthy eating is simple.

When I'm counseling patients about diet, I think of it as the "six things diet." Here are the six basic things that the earliest humans had to choose from to eat: fish, fowl (chicken, turkey, etc.), beef, fruits, vegetables, and water. This form of eating is known as the Paleo diet. There are many good books out there about eating Paleo. If you are ever having doubts as to what you are about to eat, ask yourself if it falls into one of these six categories. In its simplest form, this is healthy eating. If all you ever ate were organic fish, chicken, beef, fruits, vegetables, and water, I guarantee you would never have to worry about most of the diseases or sicknesses we've talked about thus far. Chances are you would not be overweight, lacking energy, or getting sick all the time. Clearly, eating food in its natural form is the way to go.

If you would take my word for it and only consume these six things for the rest of your life, your health would improve dramatically, your energy would soar, your lean muscle mass would increase, and so would your endurance, your libido, and just about every other marker of good health. I could literally end the chapter right here, and you'd have all the info you need on how to eat healthy. The reality is that very few people would take that and run with it, so I'll continue.

Healthy Eating Basics 101

When I educate people about weight loss and nutrition, I frequently recognize the lack of knowledge that most people have about food. I guarantee you that my nine-year-old son Nolan could make more sense out of a food label than most adults. For example, I often hear comments like this: "Johnny gets all of his protein because he eats his veggies every day." No kidding. I'm not trying to make fun of anyone or make you feel bad, but veggies aren't a primary source of protein. I hope you know that. So I'm going to explain to you in the simplest terms possible, the way I do in my seminars, about the three macronutrients: *protein, carbohydrates,* and *fats.*

Protein: If it walks, swims, or has feathers, it is a protein. Basically, if it comes from an animal, it is a protein. (i.e., eggs, beef, chicken, turkey, salmon, tuna, and cheeses)

Carbohydrates: If it grows on a tree or in the ground, it is a carb (i.e., potatoes, pasta, bread, fruits, veggies, oats, and, of course, sugars).

There are two kinds of carbs: simple and complex.

1. *Simple carbs* These are very easily and quickly digested to give you quick energy. However, they also cause strong fluctuations in insulin and will cause you to store body fat. Fruit, fruit juices, sugary drinks, alcohol, candy, and almost all processed foods are simple carbs. The types of food that contain simple carbs, such as potato chips, soda, etc., are highly toxic and should be avoided. Generally, limit your simple carbs as much as possible.

   Simple carbs are a major factor in blood sugar problems. If you have blood sugar issues, it is almost certain that you have a problem with simple carbohydrates.

Note: Many people don't know what the term *processed food* means. Just think of it this way: if it comes in a box or a bag, it's processed food.

2. *Complex carbs* These take longer to digest and contain more vitamins and fiber. Because they are slow digesting, they provide a more consistent energy source and are better for your blood sugar. Complex carbs are found in grains and vegetables and are much healthier than their counterparts. It should be noted though that many people have food sensitivities to grains.

Fats: Healthy fats are essential to a healthy body. Your brain, spinal cord, and all your cell membranes are composed of fat. Despite the fear and ignorance that is out there about eating dietary fat, it is a critically necessary component of healthy eating. Good fats come from sources like avocado, fish oil, hazelnut, almonds, flax seed and olive oil, just to name a few.

For the last few decades, we have been told that eating dietary fat causes you to be fat and also causes heart disease, high cholesterol, and the like. I am telling you that is an old, outdated theory. While I certainly don't recommend that you go around eating sticks of butter and sixteen-ounce steaks every day, dietary fat is not the enemy. I'll explain what the enemy is in just a few paragraphs.

The following is a list of recommended **Return to Health foods**. (It is assumed that all foods listed below are prepared in a healthy manner, such as grilling or broiling. No deep fried preparation should be used.)

Protein	Carbohydrates	Fats
Lean, organic beef	Sweet potato, baked potato	Avocados
Chicken breast	Steamed brown rice	Extra-virgin olive oil
Salmon (fresh, wild)	Steamed wild rice	Coconut milk, oil, etc.

Organic free-range eggs	Low-sugar oatmeal	Flaxseed
Tuna	Barley	Walnuts
Organic lean ground turkey	Low-glycemic fruits like apples, plums, apricots, peaches, pears, cherries and berries	Almonds
Turkey breast	Bananas in moderation	Pecans
Low-fat cottage cheese	grapes	Most fresh fish
Halibut (fresh, wild)	beans	Fish oil supplementation Omega-3
Orange Roughy	Vegetables like broccoli, asparagus, cauliflower, zucchini, squash, onion, spinach, artichoke, green beans, mushrooms, and peppers	
Lean ham	Greek yogurt	
Sea bass	Gluten-free breads, in moderation	
Snapper	Salad makings, like lettuce, tomato, cucumber, etc.	

If you review this chart in detail, you will see that every item on the list, except for gluten-free bread, fits into the "six things diet" regimen that I spoke of earlier. In its simplest form, this is healthy eating. People often complain that when you eat healthy, there isn't much to choose from. Really? You could easily make about a thousand different meals from the items on this list. And consider this. In all of the food diaries that I analyze, there is little variety in most people's eating regimens. The majority of people don't have a wide range of different kinds of food that they eat on a daily basis. They eat the same things over and over again, and it is usually total crap. I'll be willing to bet that if you did a seven-day food diary yourself, you'd find that you eat pretty much the same thing multiple times throughout the week, and your meals are probably the same from week to week as well.

My point: don't get caught in the negative pattern of "There isn't anything to eat when you eat healthy." What people really mean when they say that is there isn't any junk food on the list.

My Confession

As I sit here writing this, I consider myself to be an authority on what true health really is. That said, I would confess to you that I love pizza, french fries, ice cream, Starbuck's coffee, chips and dip, and lots of different desserts. By the way, my wife is a Le Cordon Bleu–trained pastry chef, and she's awesome at it! Here's the deal: I consume those things very sparingly. How sparingly, you wonder? I eat pizza maybe three times per year. I eat french fries maybe twice a year. And just because my wife is an unbelievable pastry chef doesn't mean that I sit around eating pastries all day long. Neither does she. She's approaching her fortieth birthday, has had three children, and has an incredible physique! What can I say? I love it!

I also like to have a glass of wine or a cocktail, so if you see me out at a restaurant having a drink, don't cry, "Hypocrite." One rule of healthy eating that has stood the test of time is moderation. It's not the stuff that you do once in a while that kills you; it's the stuff you do all the time. The problem lies in the fact that most people's idea of moderation is different from mine. A good example is that many American families have pizza night once per week. Eating pizza fifty-two times a year isn't moderation, but most people believe it is. They probably think, "Well, I *only* eat pizza once a week." Perception is everything, I guess.

I know that the healthy-eating purists out there will burn me in effigy for the above paragraphs. There are people who never, ever stray from a healthy-eating regimen, and I commend them for that. I am happy eating a very healthy diet about 97.8 percent of the time. I do like to live a little. Whether you end up being a purist or more like me is something you will have to figure out for yourself, but I recommend that you try to at least eat as healthy as I do. Now that you know the basics, I'm going to tell you how I do it.

Eating Healthy for Life

Obviously, we want to ingest healthy food so that we can provide our bodies with the proper nutrition it needs in the way of vitamins, minerals, and macronutrients.

But there is a much larger game going on here than meets the eye when it comes to how we eat. That larger game is the control of various hormones in our body. This may sound judgmental, but if you lined ten people up in front of me whom I'd never met before, I could tell you pretty accurately what kind of food they eat, how much of it they eat, and when they eat it, just by looking at them. No, it's not an old parlor trick. The fact of the matter is that predictable things happen to the body when you eat certain foods.

I've read countless books on nutrition and have either read or skimmed through the majority of the popular diet books that are on the market. One thing that many of them have in common is the painstaking detail they use to explain the effects of many of the fat-storing and fat-burning hormones in the body and other details of biochemistry. While this is good information to know and interesting if you are a biochemist or physician, I believe that these complicated explanations are one reason that many people reading such books fail with the diets offered by them. I have seen some recommendations in various health books that I have wanted to try myself, but the instructions and steps to implement them were so complicated and time consuming that I said, "Forget it."

I said all that to say this: let's keep this simple. As I see it, only one hormone needs to be addressed when talking about healthy eating, and that is insulin. It doesn't matter whether you are perfectly healthy or sick as a dog; this hormone needs to be under control for you to live a long, happy, healthy, and pain-free life. And if you keep insulin in check, all of the other fat-burning and fat-storing hormones will fall into place. Simple, right?

Well, how we control it is just as simple. You control insulin levels by eating smaller meals that have a balance of healthy proteins and carbohydrates and by keeping sugar intake low. Does it get any simpler than that? Sure doesn't. It's very simple. The beauty of it is that by controlling insulin, you also control blood sugar. This is why we are so proficient in getting Type II Diabetics back to a normal life. And just like we discussed earlier, having your blood sugar under control is an absolute must in overcoming chronic sickness and disease. With that being said, there is one point that I really need to drive home. *Sugar is public enemy number one!*

Let me take you back a few years. Back in the early 80s, a very popular idea was that eating dietary fat was what caused you to be fat. Along came a company called Snack Wells, and the "low fat" and "non-fat" food craze was born. They were marketing all sorts of fat-free foods, like ice cream and cookies and other kinds of junk. People bought into this *big time*. No pun intended. These foods flew off the shelves of grocery stores all over America; people believed that they could "have their cake and eat it too," so to speak. Guess what happened? Our country got fatter!

Then we moved into the 90s, and suddenly the new research showed that carbohydrates were making us fat, so along came the "low carb" and "no carb" food craze. Just like a decade earlier, those foods flew off the shelves faster than stores could stock them. People bought into this idea too, and even though the low-carb craze was more on the right track than the low-fat craze, America again got fatter!

Well, the reason is because even though the food companies had found a way to chemically alter their products so that they contained less fat or fewer carbs, the foods were still just empty, processed calories. In the case of most of the fat-free stuff, manufacturers improved the flavor by adding more sugar and carbs. The low-carb foods became even more chemically dangerous due to the fact that most of them are altered by adding aspartame or sucralose. It should be noted also that all of this started in the early 80s, and since then the increase of cancer in this country has been on a rampage, with no end in sight.

The marketing of these products as healthy foods is very deceptive— and powerful, especially if you haven't taken the time to educate yourself about what real health is. When I ask people how they eat,

I frequently get responses such as, "I eat healthy, doc. I eat mostly low-fat and low-carb foods." When I hear this I immediately know that the person I am talking to needs some serious food counseling.

Public Enemy Number One

Back to the sugar discussion. This is one concept you absolutely must get. It's critical that you do.

Sugar Point #1: When you ingest sugar, you stimulate the release of insulin. When this happens, a cascade effect takes place that causes all of your fat-storing hormones to work overtime and all of your fat-burning hormones to take a vacation. Think of an overweight person at the gym working her ass off on a treadmill every day for two years who still hasn't lost a pound. You know that person does not have a grip on insulin—insulin has a grip on them.

Sugar Point #2: There is no substance you can consume that will cause more inflammation in your body than sugar. Sugar inflames all the tissues and cells in your body. If you suffer from any type of chronic pain syndrome, autoimmune condition, cancer, or chronic health problem, it is absolutely paramount that you get a handle on the sugar issue!

Sugar Point #3: Sugar is in just about everything you eat nowadays. It is responsible for the astronomical rise that our country has seen in type II diabetes and a major player in the development of cancer and heart disease. Cancer cells absolutely love sugar. They feed off of it and grow. Interestingly, oncologists rarely tell their patients to lower their sugar intake.

Sugar Point #4: When I talk about sugar, I am not only referring to the white sweet stuff. Simple carbohydrates are also included when I use the term *sugar*. So anything that comes in a box or a bag is part of Public Enemy Number One.

Sugar Point #5: While fruit has many great health benefits, it is loaded with fructose, which is the hardest type of sugar for your body to process. Fructose also causes the liver to be sluggish and interferes with regular breakdown of food. Lastly, fructose will quickly raise insulin levels, so it is okay to eat fruit, but choose low-sugar fruits in limited quantities.

We have always been taught that eating saturated fats causes high cholesterol and heart disease. The reality is that our body was designed for saturated fats to flow through our arteries like any other food type we eat. High sugar intake causes the interior walls of your arteries to become inflamed and "sticky." That inflammation and "stickiness" inside your arteries will grab onto the saturated fats and cholesterol flowing through, which will lead to plaque build-up and artery blockage. Did you really catch what I'm saying there? It's the inflammation within the arteries from eating sugar and simple carbs that causes the cholesterol to stack up. This is another prime example of how our country is stuck in an old way of thinking and largely ignorant of the actual process that causes the problems.

If you're asking yourself why you haven't heard this before and why your doctor hasn't explained it to you this way, you're not alone. It's a long answer, but I'll give you the short version in two parts.

1. Most medical doctors receive very little formal education in nutrition. That's not an insult; it's just a fact of life.

2. Pharmaceutical companies make billions and billions of dollars selling you high cholesterol and high blood pressure drugs, so why should they tell you that sugar intake is what's causing your arteries to plug up?

Here's the point: If you want to live a long, healthy life you must stop ingesting food that is loaded with sugar and simple carbohydrates. If you're currently suffering from any type of chronic health condition, you must get control of this. I could literally write ten more pages just on this subject and explain it to you in a hundred other ways. It's that serious.

What about Artificial Sweeteners?

Glad you asked. This topic really strikes a nerve with me, so listen carefully. Stay away from pink, blue, and yellow. That means Sweet-n-Low, NutraSweet (aspartame), and Splenda (sucralose). When I say stay away from these things, I mean stay away from them like they are the plague. These are three of the most highly toxic foods ever allowed into our food chain.

If you need an artificial sweetener, I recommend that you use Truvia. At the time of this writing, everything I have learned about Truvia indicates that it is natural and there are no side effects. By contrast, aspartame and sucralose are synthetic, chemically toxic substances. Currently, there is an artificial sweetener on the rise called Neotame. Not many people have heard about it yet, but mark my words, Neotame is a bad boy! Stay away from it. Remember, we want to stay as close to God-created foods as we can.

The Easiest Explanation of Healthy Eating That You'll Ever See

I believe the nutrition principles that I preach in my practice are not only scientifically sound but also practical for everyday life. While the information I deliver to my patients has evolved over the years, these basic principles have stood the test of time. That is important, because if a diet or healthy-eating regimen frequently changes, then it is nothing more than a fad.

Over the years I have devised a very simplified regimen of healthy eating that I prescribe for my patients. Here it is:

- **Eat 5 to 6 small meals per day.** Try to evenly space them at relatively the same time each day. Each meal should be evenly balanced with protein, complex carbohydrates, and fat. This is simple. Just pick foods off of the chart that I provided. If you are overweight, this step is especially crucial to you.

- **Keep sugar to a minimum**. Ideally, you should eat somewhere between fifteen and twenty-five grams of sugar per day. In the book *Bellyfat Cure*, Jorge Cruise states that the average American consumes 189 grams of sugar per day! That's forty-seven teaspoons! If you stay between fifteen and twenty-five grams, you'll keep your insulin levels in check.

- **Keep carbohydrates to a minimum.** When counting grams of carbs on food labels, only count total carbs. Don't worry about the breakdowns below the total carbs. For our purposes, total carbs is all we're worried about. I'd like you to keep your carbs between 120 and 140 grams per day, divided over five small meals. Obviously you don't want to eat all 120 grams at one meal. You really have to watch breads and pastas. You will also want to replace regular pastas with gluten-free pastas.

- **Watch your condiments.** Ketchups, salsas, and salad dressings are loaded with sugar. You must become good at seeking out sugar in foods where you wouldn't suspect it.

- **Avoid excessive portions.** Common sense goes a long way here. Use intelligent portion control. Typically, portions no larger than the size of your hand will serve you well.

- **Remember the "six things."** When all else fails, remember the six things that early humans ate: beef, chicken, fish, fruits, vegetables, and water. Stick with that list, and you'll be golden.

The one thing I really want you to remember is that eating healthy means a lifetime commitment to being healthy. I don't like the idea of a "diet" because it implies a beginning and an ending. When you are committed to eating healthy, there is no end to it. You do it forever.

Daniel was a 57-year-old man who came to me for help with weight loss. His story went much deeper than needing to lose weight though. When I met him he was a Type II Diabetic. His daily blood sugar readings were in the high 300's, which is astronomical. He was on over a hundred units of insulin per day as well as several other medications. In addition, he suffered from neck pain, low back pain and chronic fatigue among many other health aberrations. After being under my care for only a few months he had lost over sixty pounds, twenty inches off of his waist and was down to ten units per day of insulin. Furthermore, his daily blood sugar readings were in the 90's, where they should be, he was going to the gym everyday to work out and his aches and pains were gone. His diabetes doctor was astounded, as he had been going to their clinic for years with no improvement. At last check up, his doctor told him he would soon be able to get off of his insulin. This goes to show that when you apply the appropriate measures to a health problem, you can completely turn your life around!

Vitamins and Supplements

As a natural healthcare doctor, I am greatly in favor of the use of vitamins and supplements. It is in fact a foundation of my practice. That being said, I believe that many people are taking an excessive amount of supplements that they don't need. This seems to be particularly true for people who suffer from chronic health problems. It is not uncommon for me to meet patients that are on twelve different medications and also taking fifteen different vitamins. In those cases I will usually wean them off of all their supplements and start over.

One thing that very few people are aware of is the fact that some supplements can throw the balance of your immune system off. As discussed earlier, your immune system has two sides: Th1 and Th2. In people who are dealing with autoimmune problems, the Th1/Th2 system has become out of balance. Some supplements can further throw this system out of balance and create more problems for the patient. This is why I think it is reckless to just start taking every supplement that you read about as being good for you. Check with your natural healthcare physician first.

In my opinion, most people need to take a multivitamin, vitamin C, vitamin D, fish oil and minerals. Those are the basics. Beyond that I really believe people should either undergo nutritional testing or a thorough assessment by a natural health physician before getting into additional types of supplements.

The quality of supplements and vitamins you take is important. I hate to say it, but vitamins that you buy in a store are not good quality. Most of them have very low absorption rates and are loaded with excipients. Excipients are toxic additions to supplements that manufacturers use because they are cheaper. While a certain supplement may be doing something beneficial for you, it is all for naught if you are building a toxic load in your body every time you take them. The most common excipients are magnesium stearate, talcum powder and "natural flavors", which is usually MSG. There are very few sources for top quality supplements. You usually need buy from a physician to get good supplements. I recommend that you consult with a natural healthcare physician to find the best supplements for you. To learn about how you can get a proper assessment or more about vitamins, please visit our website at www.robkuhn.com.

Food Sensitivities and Allergies

Food sensitivities and allergies are a major problem in our country. If you suffer from chronically poor health, there is a good chance you have food sensitivities that need to be addressed. I cannot even begin to emphasize how important this is. Even for something like chronic joint pain, get checked for food sensitivities. The most common offenders are gluten, dairy, eggs, and soy. In the chapter on detox, I said it was imperative that you detox your gut and liver if you suffer from a chronic health problem. Likewise, it is imperative that you get checked for food sensitivities if you have a chronic health problem. The proper approach to food sensitivities can literally change your life.

I had a male patient in his late forties come to see me last year. He felt as if though his life were totally coming off the tracks. This gentleman kept himself in great shape and was very physically fit. Despite that, he had no energy, chronic pain, shortness of breath, anxiety and several other health challenges. He had been going to his primary care doctor for years trying to figure out the problem.

The first thing I did was run a food sensitivity panel on him. It turned out that he was sensitive to eggs, dairy and gluten. We immediately got him off all of those foods and within just a couple of weeks he said that he felt better than he had since being a teenager. That is the power of functional medicine!

The food chain in our country is becoming more damaged by the day. The onset of GMOs (genetically modified food) has altered the face of nutrition. While the FDA will never admit it, these foods are worsening the health of Americans every day. I don't have space in this book to cover this topic in detail, but I highly recommend you research it for yourself. You will be appalled at what you find.

I feel it is my civic duty to give you the following prophecy. In twenty years from now, we will look back and understand that wheat has been a cause of sickness, disease, and early death in our country. American wheat has been so genetically compromised that the human body cannot properly digest it. Even if you do not have gluten sensitivity, you should never eat wheat. That includes bread, pasta, pastries, or anything made from flour. My wife has celiac disease, and before we discovered her illness, wheat was wrecking her life. I highly recommend you read the book *Wheat Belly*, by William Davis, MD.

The Big Tip

I recommend that you completely and totally eliminate wheat and dairy from your diet for a period of one month and pay attention to the changes in your health. When I say completely and totally, I mean completely. Not a crumb. Not a drop. For some people, this could be the biggest tip in the book. I can tell you that a large number of people will see dramatic improvements in their health. As a matter of fact, some people with chronic conditions will see such drastic changes that they may feel as though they no longer have the problem.

It is important to understand that you may have other food sensitivities that may need to also be addressed. The only way to know exactly what food sensitivities you have is to undergo the proper testing. It's very rare when someone comes into my office and they have already been tested for food sensitivities. If they have, 99% of the time they have had a skin prick test. That test is totally obsolete and I always consider it to be invalid. Many times I will run the food sensitivity panel that we use through Cyrex Labs, and I will find numerous sensitivities that the skin prick test did not pick up. I do consider Cyrex to be the gold standard.

Just Remember

If you stick to this kind of eating regimen day in and day out for your entire life, you will dramatically improve your chances of being healthy. You will experience improvements in mental clarity, sleep, energy, libido, stamina, and overall well-being. If you are overweight, applying this regimen to your life and sticking to it faithfully will help you lose weight so fast it will make your head spin. If you suffer from chronic pain and/or fatigue, you may see major improvements in your quality of life. Quite simply, healthy eating will change your life.

Another great aspect of committing to this type of lifestyle is that your children will grow up with good nutrition habits that will stay with them forever. I am very proud of the fact that our twenty-year-old son Alex eats an incredibly clean diet, even though he is now living on his own. He has followed our lead, further educated himself, and really knows how to eat healthy. His good fitness and nutrition habits have landed him a modeling contract with a major New York agency. I feel good knowing that he will carry those habits with him for his entire life, and as a result, he is much less likely to become a healthcare statistic.

Action Steps:

- Make a commitment to healthy eating

- Achieve an optimal pH of 6.4 – 7.0

- Remember the six things, beef, fowl, fish, fruits, vegetables and water

- Stay away from artificial sweeteners

- Eat multiple small meals per day

- Decrease your sugar and simple carbohydrates

- Stop taking vitamins you don't need

- If your health is chronically poor or you have autoimmune issues, you must get checked for food sensitivities

- Eliminate wheat and dairy for a period of one month and track your progress

Chapter 7

Exercise Is For Life

> You simply cannot escape this reality: Your body is the epicenter of your universe. You go nowhere without it. It is truly the temple of your mind and your soul. If it is sagging, softening, and aging rapidly, other aspects of your life will soon follow suit.
>
> —Bill Phillips, *Body for Life*

The quote that I chose to open this chapter with comes from the bestselling book *Body for Life* by Bill Phillips. I read that book years ago and have never forgotten this statement. There is one sentence in that paragraph which I absolutely love: "your body is the epicenter of your universe." This is a powerful statement and 100 percent accurate. Think about it. It doesn't matter what you want to accomplish in your life, what you want to do, or where you want to go, you need a vibrant, healthy body to do it in. Period!

Over the years, I have all too often seen people whose bodies are breaking down who haven't even given a second thought to exercising in decades. In fact, it has been my experience that the percentage of people who actually include exercise as a regular, consistent part of their lives is very small. What I mean by regular exercise is regularly scheduled exercise routines that you keep up with week after week, year after year. In my opinion, the person who gets into exercising every few months and sticks with it for a week or two doesn't qualify as someone who exercises regularly; nor does the person who exercises once a week. Sorry, but that's reality.

Everyone I have known who has just started back into exercising proclaims that he or she feels much better when working out regularly. Well, if you know it makes you feel better, why wouldn't you keep it up? Excuses, that's why! If you were being really honest with yourself, wouldn't you say that's true?

Excuses, Excuses!

"I don't have enough time" is the most common excuse people use for not exercising. Early in my career I attended a very intense personal development camp. One of the activities was a time assessment drill where we accounted for every moment of our day. For me, the results of this were stunning. Even as an extremely busy person with three kids and a business to run, I was surprised to find how much time I wasted in my day, and I don't like wasting time. The reality is that you probably do have time to exercise. If you find out otherwise, then you need to get up an hour earlier every day.

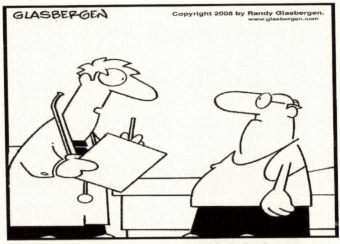

"What fits your busy schedule better,
exercising one hour a day or being
dead 24 hours a day?"

If it seems that I'm being a little insistent about not making excuses and finding time to exercise, it's because this subject is that important. Failure to exercise will set into motion numerous breakdown processes in the human body. Conversely, maintaining a regular exercise routine in your life will create an abundance of health in all areas. Below is a short list of benefits that exercise provides the human body.

- Improves heart function
- Lowers blood pressure
- Reduces body fat
- Elevates bone mass
- Prevents brain degeneration
- Improves learning
- Slows and reverses the aging process
- Decreases total and LDL cholesterol
- Elevates HDL (good) cholesterol

- Raises energy levels

- Enhances and balances hormone production

- Aids sleep

- Increases stress tolerance and promotes stress release

- Eliminates toxins

- Reduces depression

- Can control, reverse or prevent diabetes

- Decreases risk of injury to joints, muscles, and ligaments

- Speeds up metabolism

- Protects against falls

- Increases sex drive

- Helps prevent dementia and Alzheimer's

This is a brief list of benefits, but if you read between the lines, there is a much bigger picture involved here. Can you see it? According to the above list of benefits, regular exercise reduces or eliminates the need for about seven of the most over-prescribed, over-marketed, and over-hyped medications on the market: i.e., high blood pressure meds, high cholesterol meds, antidepressants, weight-loss drugs, erectile dysfunction drugs, sleeping pills, and osteoporosis meds, to name a few. So basically, if everyone exercised on a regular basis, we'd be a much healthier nation, and the debt that piles up every year due to medical expenses would be drastically lowered. Sounds like a good idea to me.

The Hottest Thing in Healthcare

Over the last several years all things related to anti-aging have become quite the rage in healthcare. You'll see products such as vitamins, skin creams, and pharmaceutical drugs touting their respective anti-aging qualities. We are constantly inundated with advertising messages about looking and feeling younger. Despite being in the midst of the worst economy we've seen in our lifetime, plastic surgery centers are busier than they have ever been. You can find medical offices whose chosen field of care is anti-aging. Yes, vanity sells. There is no question about that.

As is usually the case in our society, most people try to bypass doing what should be done to remain youthful and healthy and instead try all kinds of crazy gimmicks, dangerous drugs, and even surgeries to get their lives back. Many of the so-called anti-aging clinics are nothing more than legalized steroid mills. Doctors prescribe growth hormones and steroids under the guise of "modern medicine." What is once again horribly missing is the fact that there are underlying causes for why your body may be deficient in these natural hormones. In most cases, the body is not producing the hormones at normal levels due to a problem with some other metabolic pathway in the body. Covering that problem up by prescribing hormone replacement may result in normal hormone levels on a blood test, but it further damages the body's negative feedback loop system, thus driving the malfunctioning part of the body into the danger zone.

Staying true to the major theme of this book, my goal is to help you live the longest, happiest, healthiest life possible. In order to do that, you will need to create natural anti-aging processes in the body. Regular exercise is an absolute necessity and a key component for that result.

> What lies behind us, and what lies before us, is nothing compared to what lies within us.

Your Body Is Not a 1962 Corvette!

Early 1960s Corvettes are some of my favorite classic cars. If you can find a mint condition 1962 Corvette that has been beautifully stored in a garage for decades, chances are it'll be worth a lot of money. Keeping it in the garage will prevent the sun from damaging the paint and drying out the interior. If it is rarely driven, the motor, transmission, and other moving parts will most likely maintain a nice working order, provided that it is run often enough to keep it healthy. There is also much less chance that this beautiful vehicle will be scratched or damaged in an accident if it is kept in a garage and hardly used. The bottom line is that the less you use a classic car like this, the longer it will last and the more value it will retain.

Your body is exactly the opposite. The old adage "If you don't use it, you lose it" is totally accurate when applied to the human body. The less you use your body for things other than just sitting at a desk or in front of the television, the more it will break down. When you don't exercise, your body and your muscles will quickly atrophy, which means break down and shrink. Guess what? Your heart, your lungs, and your organs are muscles! This means that when you make the choice to be lazy for days, weeks, months, and years on end, you are increasing atrophy in your organs too. Translation: you are consciously choosing to shorten your life and lower the overall quality of your life.

Consider this quote from a recent study on fitness from Dr. Vonda Wright, published in the *New York Times*:

> The changes that we've always assumed were due to aging and therefore were unstoppable seem actually to be caused by inactivity.

What Dr. Wright is saying is that we've always blamed breakdown in the body on normal aging, but the research is showing that inactivity (doing nothing, being lazy, sedentary, etc.) is the actual cause.

I am always amazed when I see people who are only in their thirties, forties, or fifties and they can't even enjoy a day at Disneyland or going Christmas shopping, because they can't be on their feet for more than an hour. Yes, I know there are people who are born with disabilities or who have encountered tragic accidents who make this their reality. I'm not talking about them, so spare me the "you're not being fair" routine. The reality is that most people who can't walk or stand for any length of time have reached that point because they have consciously chosen to treat their body like crap.

The good news is that it is never too late to turn it around. If you make the decision right now to start exercising, within three months you could be living in a totally different body! If that doesn't excite you, you should probably just put this book down and start counting the days until you die. C'mon, let's get off the couch and get going!

But Doc, I'm Too Old!

This excuse is so lame that I almost don't want to give it any attention, but unfortunately it is so frequently used that I have to. After thirteen years of practice I am still astonished at how many people come in saying, "Doc, I'm getting old." The reason it amazes me is because I commonly hear that come out of the mouths of people in their thirties and forties!

The only reason people make these asinine statements is because they have been inactive and sedentary for so long that their bodies are starting to break down. Do you want to hear the easy cure? Stop sitting on your butt and go move your body! It's really that easy. And it literally doesn't matter if you are eighty years old; you can get just as good results as someone who is in their twenties.

Did you know that people in their eighties and nineties are regularly running full marathons? Many people are familiar with Jack LaLanne and all the incredible physical feats he performed until his recent death at the age of ninety-six. (By the way, most people don't know that Jack LaLanne was a chiropractor.) Here are a few other incredible things that people are doing into old age. These come from an article in *Happy News*, which I read on Mercola.com.

- A ninety-eight-year-old woman received her tenth degree black belt in judo

- Tao Porchon-Lynch competes in ballroom dance competitions and teaches at least twelve yoga classes a week at age ninety-three

- Lew Hollander became the second eighty-year-old to complete the Ford Ironman World Championship, which consists of a 2.4-mile swim, a 112-mile bike ride, and a 26.2-mile marathon

- Allan Johnson, at age eighty, still competes in rodeo competitions

So what were your excuses for not exercising? When it comes down to it, unless you are missing some limbs or you have a heart that is so poorly functioning that your cardiologist has told you that you can never exercise, all that's left are excuses. Let's just agree to leave those in the dust and get moving, shall we?

What Are the Goals?

As I see it, there is one all-encompassing goal for exercise: to create a healthy body that will last you a lifetime. Remember, good health is not something that happens by accident, but rather, it is something that you create. Exercising is a major part of the foundation that creates excellent health. Go back and look at the short list of benefits I showed you earlier in this chapter; it encompasses just about every system in the body. Either directly or indirectly, you can connect everything on that list to the:

Cardiovascular system

Respiratory system

Endocrine system

Skeletal system

Nervous system

Lymphatic system

Integumentary system (skin)

This list pretty much makes up your whole body. There isn't a pill or potion out there that can affect each of these systems in such a positive manner. The best part is that regular exercise can make you feel absolutely incredible.

Why do you think there is such a huge problem with depression in our society today compared to a hundred years ago? While depression can be a complicated issue to solve, looking at it from an exercise perspective can really give us some clues. A hundred years ago, the majority of people in our country had a very lively physical life. There weren't a whole lot of jobs out there that required a person to sit all day long. Most people did a plethora of physical work to maintain their households, wash their clothes and prepare their food. Vehicles were in limited supply; most people walked or rode horses everywhere they went. There was no such thing as television, video games, or computers, so people relied on physical activity to entertain themselves. Having such a consistent flow of physical activity allowed the endocrine system, which controls your hormones, to be in top working order. People experienced regular releases of neurotransmitters and endorphins, which make your brain and body feel good.

Let's compare that to present-day life. In 2012, more than 75 percent of the American work force sits all day long at work. We have machines to do our dishes and clean our clothes. Sadly, most people microwave the majority of their meals. We have access to every kind of motorized transportation available, and people make sure that they park as close to the building they are visiting as possible. People are addicted to television, video games, and the Internet, so they sit all day and all night long. The endocrine system in present-day Americans is not being stimulated the way that it was a hundred years ago, so we don't have the same patterns of neurotransmitter and endorphin release as we did back then. No wonder so many people are depressed!

Now, realize that I haven't even talked about nutrition, stress, and medications in regard to depression yet. I just want you to get a good sense of how powerful and important exercising is as it relates to one single health condition.

Take Control of Your Life

One of the major functions of this book is to help you reclaim your life. If you haven't noticed, I'd like nothing more than for you to kick your medications to the curb and never have to rely on them again. Consistent, regular exercise can help you take back control of your life. When I was sick with the mold, I did my best to exercise as much as I could. I will tell you that there were days when I just couldn't. It wasn't an excuse. Because my lungs were inflamed and I could barely breathe, I literally couldn't. But every day that I could muster the energy and the breath to do it, I exercised.

I went out for runs, lifted weights, or did yoga when I felt absolutely horrible. It was rough, but whenever I finished the exercise I felt empowered. I can clearly recall thinking that if I could still exercise, then I could eventually pull through. That is the way that I want you to think! I want you to realize that you are in control of your life. If you can do even a little bit of exercise, you can pull through your health challenges. You must believe that! Forget what everyone else is telling you.

You have fibromyalgia? You have hypothyroidism? You have type II diabetes? You have chronic migraine headaches? You better take control of your life now! Because if you wait and let your doctors make your decisions for you, you will continue the downhill slide toward misery. Sorry if I'm the first to tell you that, but it's true. It astounds me when patients come to my office who are in states of chronically bad health, have been on multiple medications for years, and are clearly getting worse, and yet they still act as if they cannot do anything without asking their doctor's permission first. The same doctor who has gotten them nowhere, mind you. Stop it! Please, take control of your life now before it's too late.

Exercising is a great place to start. It will give you the power to feel like you can do anything and help you to realize that you can break through challenges. If you don't have a regular routine of exercise, you've got to get started now.

What Kind of Exercise Should You Do?

There are numerous directions you can go in.

First of all, you won't find a workout routine with pictures in my book. Why? Well, first of all, this isn't an exercise book. Secondly, it has been my experience that if people are inspired by a book to work out, very rarely will they take that book to the gym and utilize the pictures in the book to help them work out. In most cases, people are going to do whatever kind of exercise that they most enjoy or enlist the help of a personal trainer, so a workout routine isn't necessary in this book.

It is crucial that you develop a program that provides *both* resistance training and cardiovascular exercise.

- **Resistance training** (also known as strength training). This training is designed to develop strength in your muscles by utilizing bands or weights to create an opposition of force. As you age, resistance training is critical for maintaining a strong musculoskeletal system and adequate bone mass and for controlling body fat. This type of training should be utilized by people of all ages. I have noticed a common thread in people over the age of seventy-five that are in excellent health and great shape; they always lift weights.

- **Cardiovascular exercise** (also known as cardio). Cardio is important to maintaining optimally functioning cardiovascular, pulmonary, and circulatory systems. Regular cardiovascular exercise has also been shown to increase mental health and improve stamina. Cardiovascular exercise includes walking, jogging, cycling, swimming, and using treadmill, stairmaster, and elliptical machines, just to name a few.

I believe it's important that you do the kind of exercise that is most pleasing to you. If you know you like swimming, do that. If you know you enjoy walking, do it. If you know you like to play tennis, do it. Here's the thing—you need to mix it up, you need to schedule it, and you need to keep it consistent.

Here are some simple recommendations.

1. Start by building a foundation. If you haven't exercised in a long time, start by going for a short walk. Fifteen to twenty minutes will do. Try doing this at least three days per week for a few weeks. If you have no problem with it, try doing it every other day, then every day. When you are working out at least five days per week, I'd say that you have a good foundation under you. I've had patients with COPD or heart conditions who literally started building their foundation by taking daily walks from their front door to the mailbox. You do what you need to do for success.

2. If you have fibromyalgia, arthritis, or any chronic pain syndrome, try yoga. It is a phenomenal workout for fibro patients. Once you get in the groove and you do it consistently, your body will love you for it. Remember this: the best thing for chronic pain is movement. When you are sedentary, your pain levels will be worse. There are numerous DVDs available with great yoga workouts that are easy to follow. Of course you can check with your local gym or YMCA to see if they offer beginning yoga classes. Most of them do.

3. Once you have gotten through a month of building a foundation for exercise, move up to more strenuous workouts. Try weight lifting. You can hire a personal trainer or ask the employees at your local gym about how to use equipment and what types of workouts to do. If you are the kind of person who likes to use workouts from books, there are hundreds of books out there dedicated to that one thing. As always, start light, and work your way up.

4. Once you are really rolling, if you have the gumption and the physical ability, you can work your way up to doing popular home workouts like P90X or Insanity. Bob Harper and Jillian Michaels of Biggest Loser fame also offer excellent workout videos. I have done them, and they are great. These workouts are very intense, though, so be sure you are good and ready for them before you begin.

5. Rotate your workouts. Do strength training one day, cardio the next, then maybe play tennis, and then start over. Find what works for you, and stick with it!

As I stated earlier, it was not my goal in this chapter to teach you how to exercise but to teach you why you need to exercise. Should you happen to attend one of my life-changing seminars, we will teach you some different forms of exercise. But for the purposes of this book, my goal is to build a case for exercising and get you to commit to it once and for all. Just as a lawyer tries to string together a sequence of evidence to make the jury see one side of a case, I want you to truly understand the necessity and importance of maintaining a daily, consistent exercise routine for your entire life. That's correct; I said *"daily"* and *"entire life."*

Based on everything that I have learned through a lifetime of athletics, working as a personal trainer and becoming a doctor, I am of the very strong belief that the human body functions at the highest levels and maintains the most optimal levels of health if it is exercised daily. I also know from research and clinical experiences that people who are dealing with chronic health problems see much higher recovery rates when they begin and maintain regular exercise.

If you are serious about regaining and building a life of optimal health, put together an exercise plan that suits you, and begin at once. It will be one of the best things you have ever done.

Action Steps:

- Decide that you want to be healthy for the rest of your life

- Decide which type of exercise you want to start with and begin at once: I recommend a daily walk of at least twenty minutes

- Commit to a regular schedule of exercise and stick with it

- Either sign up at a gym, get the help of a trainer, or purchase some workout DVDs to keep you rolling

Chapter 8

Less Sleep = Less Health

Each night, when I go to sleep, I die. And the next
morning, when I wake up, I am reborn.
—Mahatma Gandhi

So far, we've talked about several things that you can actively do to
overcome health challenges and catapult you to higher levels of optimal
health. You don't need to finish this book to start on those. "Begin at once"
is a great policy. But now we have arrived at a subject that might be one of
the single most important things you can do for your overall health, and
that is to be inactive. I am talking about getting proper rest.

A good night's sleep is an integral part of living a healthy life. This
is a major factor in preventing disease, pain, and sickness before they
occur. It blows my mind how many patients in my community have
been to an actual sleep center to be analyzed for various conditions and
sleep disorders. Certainly, this is a big issue.

In my personal opinion, you don't need to have a lot of fancy tests run to achieve better sleep. Like most things regarding health, if something about your sleep patterns is screwed up, there are reasons for it, and medicating them away will do nothing but more damage. Don't get me wrong. If you are dealing with something that could be potentially fatal, like sleep apnea, you need to get it checked out. But do you really want to wear a Darth Vader mask on your face every night for the rest of your life? There are ways to fix these problems. Let's examine them.

What Sleep Does For You

First of all, let's talk about the restorative powers of sleep. The greatest properties of healing take place while you are sleeping. Of course, the human body is so magnificent that it has the ability to heal while you are reading this book, drinking a cup of tea and petting your dog all at the same time. But the powerful restoration happens at night while you are in La-La Land.

Getting proper amounts of rest is beneficial for blood pressure, stress reduction, energy levels, hormone production and balance, cognitive thinking, proper brain function, healing, ideal immunity, and an optimally functioning digestive system. Conversely, if you are not getting proper rest, all of those systems will be out of balance and prone to malfunction. So in the interest of truly taking charge of your health, let's analyze which medications could probably be decreased or thrown away if people were getting proper rest.

- Blood pressure meds
- Antidepressants
- Anti-anxiety drugs
- Acid reflux drugs
- Antibiotics
- Antivirals
- Drugs for chronic fatigue

121

This is a small portion of some of the drug categories people take to combat illnesses and conditions that could be greatly minimized or eliminated by a good night's sleep. I am always baffled when people begin a new medication or procedure and don't ask themselves what the plan will be for the rest of their lives. I mean really—are you going to take sleeping pills for the rest of your life?

I can already hear the objections. "Well, Dr. Kuhn, the problem is that we can't get to sleep or stay asleep, so what do we do about that?" Well, unfortunately, most people take Ambien, Nytol, or some other sleeping pill that only compounds the problem. Don't think that just because the pill makes you go to sleep that it is helping you, because it's not … it is in fact making your sleeping problem worse and forcing you to become addicted to the drug in order to sleep. Pretty ingenious plan by the drug manufacturers, wouldn't you say?

Once they got their sleep cycles back on track, many patients over the years have seen their chronic pain syndromes and health issues decrease and/or disappear. So what does a good night's sleep do for you? Well, everything!

Why Can't You Sleep?

Let's revisit this idea that you can't get to sleep or stay asleep. It's become predictable to me to hear how many of my patients tell me that they have problems sleeping. The reason it doesn't surprise me anymore is because I've seen it so often. I take care of chronic-condition patients in my practice, and their sleeping cycles are always distorted.

As I see it, there are two causes for why people have difficulty sleeping. The catch-22 is that these causes compound each other and keep the vicious cycle going round and round. The two different categories I'm referring to are mental and physiological.

Mental. There are a few ways that this category of sleep disturbance presents.

- The person with the classic "I'm a night owl" mindset. In this line of thinking, the person is convinced that he was just born to stay up late. He can't fall asleep until he's watched enough TV, surfed the Internet, read magazines, or something similar. These people will argue until they are blue in the face that there is nothing they can do about their sleep habits because they are night owls. I am intimately familiar with this type because I was in this category for much of my life. Now, I agree with Anthony Robbins. I remember reading in one of his books (I'm paraphrasing here) that all people have to do is decide that being a night owl is a choice and not something they are cursed with, and they can change it instantly. The day I read that I stopped being a night owl.

I had a patient a few years ago who was approximately fifty-five years old and had been dealing with chronic pain for years. She was from a fairly well to do family, always dressed well, and had a nice, friendly demeanor. Upon examination I noticed that one of her main problems was that she was a smoker. If you smoke, you're not healing from anything and that's just the way it goes. Your body will be oxygen depleted, and you are in a steady downhill slide until the end of your life. But other than that, I really didn't notice anything spectacular. I began working on her, and we saw decent improvements but nothing really to brag about. Roughly a month into her care, I asked her about her sleeping habits. She responded by telling me she recorded all of her daytime soap operas and watched them between the hours of midnight and four o'clock in the morning. I asked her why, and she said it's because she was a night owl; she watched soaps at night so she had something to do.

Can you imagine staying up all night long every single night by choice? I can envision this lady sitting in her house, smoking cigarettes and watching television for four hours straight every single night, completely wreaking havoc on her circadian rhythms and destroying any possible benefits of the healing powers of sleep. I told her that she needed to change that lifestyle or she would never be free from pain. It was about that time that she stopped coming to see me. Some people do not want to hear the truth. I would bet any money that today she is probably on several different medications, still staying up all night, and still having chronic pain.

Another way people mentally sabotage their sleep is by laying awake and obsessing over everything that is going on in their lives. This applies to an overwhelming number of people in our society. You probably don't need me to tell you that no amount of obsessing about your problems will solve them, especially in the middle of the night.

***Physiological*:** There are several physiological reasons why a person might not be able to sleep. For the purposes of this book, I will focus on two. Remember, the whole purpose of this book is to help you overcome chronically bad health and to achieve optimal levels of health. In my practice I take care of some seriously sick people. I frequently see one or both of the following issues, so let's talk about them.

1. **Adrenal Problems.** I spoke about the adrenal glands in chapter 3. They are your stress glands. When a person reaches a point of poor health, the adrenal glands will start to go awry ... you can count on it. When they do go haywire, the resulting problems with cortisol rhythms will destroy any chances you have of getting a good night's rest. You will either have problems getting to sleep, or staying asleep, or both. When a patient tells me that they don't sleep well, the adrenal glands are the first thing I test. I said this before in chapter 3, but I think it's worth repeating: the adrenals are rarely ever checked in a medical office. To doctors like me, its just common sense to check the adrenals with a chronic health issue.

2. **Neurotransmitter Problems.** Neurotransmitters are chemicals in your brain. While they have numerous functions, they must be in good balance for you to be able to sleep well. If you are having neurotransmitter problems, it is very likely that you will have difficulty sleeping. This is especially true of serotonin and dopamine. Inflammatory processes, blood sugar problems, nutritional deficiencies, immunity issues, and

stress can throw off your neurotransmitter balance. It is very popular in natural healthcare circles to prescribe a melatonin supplement to help people sleep, and it works for many of them. However, I will tell you that it is a bad thing if melatonin helps you sleep. Why? Because it almost certainly means that you have a serotonin problem that needs to be fixed. Using melatonin to help you sleep will only further damage the serotonin problem. I'm not against using melatonin once in a while to help you sleep in certain situations, but daily use is not good, in my opinion. This is no different than medicating. You are only addressing a symptom (not being able to fall asleep) and not getting to the cause (serotonin problem).

As it turns out, I always address the adrenal glands and neurotransmitters in my practice because in chronic-condition patients they are frequently a problem. If you want to really take your health to the next level, these need to be checked. From a physiological standpoint, if you get these two areas under control you will see your sleep improve dramatically.

> # Your body's ability to heal is much greater than anyone has permitted you to believe.

Creating a Healthy Sleep Pattern

By now you should know how important a good night's sleep is. You should also see that the most powerful healing takes place while you are sleeping. We have discussed the more common problems with sleep; now let's talk about how to actually get a good night's rest. If you follow my steps, you will find very quickly that are you able to achieve better sleep.

First of all, it is imperative that you sleep in a position that is healthy for your spine and nervous system. I have seen more people than I can count who have created chronic pain problems by sleeping in improper positions.

When you sleep on your stomach, you break your back. It is the worst possible position for you to sleep in. Technically speaking, it is best to sleep on your back, using a cervical pillow or a very thin pillow. This will allow for the least amount of undue stress on your spine.

Now that you understand the need for proper positioning, it is important to determine if you have an adrenal or neurotransmitter problem. Visit my website and download a neurotransmitter questionnaire to find out if you have a problem in this area. I will do my best to set you up with an appropriate doctor in your area to help you resolve these problems. Whether or not you do have an adrenal or neurotransmitter problem, proceed to the next paragraph and follow my steps.

When it comes to any aspect of health, there is one concept I want you to remember: the body loves rhythm! I'll say that again: *the body loves rhythm*! This is especially true when it comes to sleep patterns. Begin to develop a pattern of going to bed and waking up at relatively close to the same time each day. Those times are up to you, but let me give you an example. I always try to go to bed at 11 pm. I don't want to lie to you and tell you that happens every night, but that is my target. To stay in a nice rhythm, I recommend that you pick a target time to go to sleep each night and try to stay within a fifteen-minute window of that bedtime each night. I go to bed most nights at 11 pm, but some nights it's 10:45pm and some nights it's 11:15pm, so I'm doing pretty good. I'm no more than fifteen minutes off, give or take.

The same holds true for waking up. I've always been an early riser, and lately I have been waking up at 5 am, as I am trying to accomplish more in my life. Staying on track with waking up at the same time each day is much easier than going to bed at the same time. Set your alarm, and when it goes off, get up. I've never understood people who are late for work because they "slept late." How excited are you about your life? Get up and get going!

On weekends, these times change for me and even become random. I love having date nights with my wife, and we have a social life, so we stay up much later on the weekends. Yes, I do sleep in on the weekends, but a late day for me is about 7:30 am. The point is, when Sunday night rolls around, I'm back on track.

As you work on establishing what time you wish to go to bed at night, keep the following in mind. Researchers say that every hour of sleep you get before midnight is worth two hours of sleep after midnight. It doesn't matter what time zone you live in, this is true. I recommend you try it. You'll find that when you are actually asleep by no later than eleven o'clock at night, you will wake up the next day feeling amazing.

Note: If you work a graveyard or swing shift, adapt this concept as best you can in your schedule; (i.e., go to bed and get up at same time each day as best you can.)

Break Your Bad Sleep Habits

Now that you've established a bed time and wake time, let's discuss something that must be talked about: the television. Although the best recommendation is to do some inspirational reading before dozing off, I do sometimes like to watch a few minutes of TV before I go to sleep. It is always something light and pleasing. Usually, it's a few minutes of catching up on scores on ESPN or an old sitcom, like *Seinfeld* or *Friends. Do not* watch the news or anything heavy, such as violent movies or shows about social problems or the like. Keep it light and short!

The next thing is to deal with all those nasty, annoying thoughts that you obsess over while laying in bed at night. When you really think about it, this is just silly. I mean, how long have you been doing that? Has it ever gotten you anywhere? Has it ever miraculously solved your problems right before you fell asleep? So why do you continue to sabotage your sleep by obsessing over these things? Just stop it!

Here is a good trick for defeating this problem. First of all, when you lay down to go to sleep, play back your entire day from the time you woke up until lying there in bed. If a negative event occurred during the day, just accept it as a learning experience. If someone wronged you, forgive him or her and realize that he or she is not perfect. If you wronged someone, forgive yourself, and make a mental note to make it right with that person the next day if possible. If something amazing happened, thank God for it and appreciate that moment, realizing that you do have good things in your life. If there is an event that is particularly pressing or stressful, just realize that you won't be able to do anything about it while you are asleep and that you will tend to it tomorrow. Here's the secret to this little drill: if you do this day in and day out, you will quickly get to the point where you will fall asleep after a minute into it. You won't even be able to recall your whole day because you will be fast asleep.

Don't drink alcohol to help yourself sleep at night. This will have a reverse effect when it begins to disrupt your neurotransmitters and blood sugar. This will also create chemical stress that will throw off your adrenal glands. Are you starting to see how this all plays in together? Like I said earlier, I can enjoy a glass of wine or a cocktail as much as anyone, but it's not a habit. I know some people would rather die than give up their wine before bed and you could even look at some European cultures and make an argument for it. But remember, I am trying to teach you how to reach the highest levels of optimal health, and daily alcohol doesn't fit in. You are much better off to have a nice cup of warm green tea.

One more thing—try to have your last meal of the day at least three hours before you go to sleep, and don't snack before bed. (This will also help you to keep fit and trim.) If your body has to work hard to digest food while sleeping, it's going to throw you off, so keep your meals far away from bedtime.

The Sleep Disrupters

I've already mentioned these, but they are worth repeating. Hei
list of the top sleep disrupters.

- Sleeping pills: yes, they are a sleep disrupter, not a sleep aid!

- Alcohol: same thing

- Eating too much before bed

- Obsessing over your life's events

- Going to sleep at a different time each day

- Negative television or sleeping with the TV on

- Adrenal and Neurotransmitter problems

Adopting some of the positive sleep habits I've described in this chapter could bridge a big gap between where your health is now and where you want it to be. Getting enough restful sleep is a critical piece of the good health puzzle. By implementing these methods immediately and steering clear of the sleep disrupters, you will soon see your health getting back on track.

Action Steps

- The body loves rhythm

- The best healing takes place while you are sleeping

- Go to bed and get up at the same time each day

- Relax with an inspirational book and a cup of green tea before bed

- Avoid sleep disrupters

- Review your day like a movie in your mind from start to finish

Chapter 9

Stress, the Three-Headed Monster

If you ask what is the single most important key to longevity,
I would have to say it is avoiding worry, stress, and tension.
And if you didn't ask me, I'd still have to say it.

—George Burns

I hate to rate these chapters in order of importance because in my opinion they are all extremely important, but this chapter is right up there at the top of the list. One of the things that I find very interesting in my practice, and in life in general, is when I come across people who say that they don't have any stress. Listen, there is only one kind of person on the planet who has no stress, and that type of person resides in a cemetery!

Fortunately, I can give you an example from someone I'm very intimate with: me! As my wife will tell you, I am a very even-keeled person, which is to say that I'm pretty consistent with my emotions.

This is not to say that I'm boring, because I'm not. If something excellent happens, I'll get as excited as anyone, but still manage to keep things in perspective. On the flip side, when the chips are down and the world seems to be crashing all around us, I'll keep my head above water. I don't let stress cause massive swings in my emotions. How I got that way, I have no idea. My mother was the ultimate worrywart, and my dad was easily excitable. Here's the point: by no means am I an emotionally perfect person. I have my good days and bad, and I'm sure my office staff, Ashley and Rebecca, will attest to that. Even though I do manage to stay even-keeled most of the time and feel as though I am very good at handling stress, I still have stress, and I would never be so flippant to say that I don't.

When patients in my office are suffering from numerous health issues or a chronic condition and say they have no stress, I know that I am dealing with someone who is in some level of denial. Being able to identify what your stressors are and understanding the different types of stress can be extremely valuable in helping you regain your health. Unless you are a Buddhist monk who has reached a level of Zen, chances are that you are probably dealing with quite a bit of stress. Accepting that and dealing with it are paramount.

Stress Kills ... Literally

It is pretty much common knowledge by now that the majority of heart attacks occur Monday morning at about 9 am. Everyone knows that this is because it is the beginning of the workweek, and most people are stressed out about their jobs. In fact, many people hate their jobs. It's been my experience that quite a bit of the working public is not happy with their vocation. So stress levels rise, the person dreads going to work, eats a crappy breakfast, gets stuck in a traffic jam on the way to the office, walks into a place that he or she hates, and, voila, has a heart attack. Yes, stress does kill.

There are more heart attacks and stress-related deaths during the holidays than any other time of the year. I don't need to tell you that although the holidays are supposed to be a joyous time, for many people they are highly stressful. The fact that researchers can pinpoint what time of the day, what day of the week, and what season of the year that most heart attacks happen gives a lot of ammunition to the idea that stress kills.

Personally, I believe that stress is the reason why my dad is no longer with us. Sadly, the last few years of my dad's life were probably the most stressful that I can recall. He retired in 2008 at the age of sixty-three after a long, successful career working for General Electric in the nuclear power division. My dad was great at what he did and very well respected in his profession. As soon as he retired, he started his own company doing the same thing he was doing for GE, only as an independent contractor, and he immediately began making a nice living at it. By that point, my dad had endured close to two decades of my mother's poor health. Dad was constantly stressed about what would happen next with my mom. In April 2008, my brother attempted suicide and spent a week in the hospital in a coma. I remember my dad telling me that seeing my brother on that ventilator in the hospital was one of the worst things that he ever experienced.

Unfortunately, two years later my mom went into the hospital on the July Fourth weekend of 2010 and never came out. She was in the ICU for six weeks before she died. My dad was by her side all day, every day. Dad was a strong man, but he would call me, crying, as we discussed what our next move was or what decisions needed to be made. My mom was on and off the ventilator; until the day she died, we kept getting reports that she was making a turnaround. The last six weeks of her life were incredibly stressful on my dad.

After her death, my dad did his duties: planning her funeral, getting her affairs taken care of, and basically putting her whole life to rest. If you've never been the one to do this, it is an amazingly exhausting and stressful process. I know, because just ninety-two days after my mom passed away, my dad woke up perfectly healthy on November 17, 2010, went to church, and on his way home had an aneurism and died. My mom was sixty-three and my dad was sixty-five. As a result of the three-headed monster called stress, they both died way too young.

Identifying the Three Kinds of Stress

If you want to reach the highest levels of optimal health, you must identify your primary stressors. I call stress the three-headed monster for a reason. We face three different kinds of stress as human beings: physical, chemical, and emotional.

Physical stress. This includes just about all the physical things that have happened to you throughout the course of your life. For some it starts at birth. Many people experience very difficult deliveries when they are born. Day one sets into motion a cascade of events that will progressively worsen over the course of their life. I will cover this in greater detail in the chapter on the nervous system.

Take into account all other forms of physical stress, such as heavy lifting, car accidents, sitting at a computer for long periods of time (which, by the way, is one of the most strenuous things you can do to your body), playing sports, sleeping in improper positions, sitting on badly designed furniture, doing yard work, being overweight, having poor posture, etc. This is just a fraction of the different types of physical stress.

Chemical stress. You may not realize it, but I've been talking about chemical stress throughout this entire book. The number one offender is eating an unhealthy diet. The majority of Americans are eating fast food, processed food, and toxin-filled food. I personally believe that most Americans really have no idea what is in the food they are eating or how preparation affects it. Surely if they were aware, they wouldn't eat it, right? These days you have to be really careful because you can go to the grocery store and try to do right by buying food in the produce section and wind up taking home food that is genetically modified (GMO). The food supply in our country is becoming unhealthier by the day, and you must educate yourself to maintain a healthy life.

The next big offender in this category is medication. *All medications are toxic!* All of them! Yet people pop them like they are health food. If you are taking medication on a regular basis, your body is chemically stressed out to the max. You must find a way to reduce or eliminate as many medications as possible. Be careful. Do this with the assistance of your doctor.

Other chemical stressors include environmental toxins like chemicals in paint, carpet, household cleaners, detergents, clothing, makeup, hair products, skin products, and hair dyes. Don't forget about excessive consumption of alcohol, illegal drugs, and cigarettes. Last but not least, are dangerous biotoxins, like black mold and Lyme's disease. Yes, chances are that your body is under a lot of chemical stress right now.

Emotional stress. We're all familiar with this one, right? Are you married? Do you have kids? Do you have a job? Do you have a boss? Then you know what emotional stress is all about. You'll usually discover that you are emotionally stressed when you fly off the handle over the smallest events, such as being cut off in traffic or your child spilling a drink at the dinner table.

As I write, with the economy so bad, war on all corners of the earth, and constant messages by drug companies that you should be taking the latest and greatest antidepressant or anti-anxiety drug, emotional stress is at an all-time high. Don't fall into that trap!

The sad thing about emotional stress is that you can actually see it. I can see it in the posture of my patients. I see it in the lines on their faces, the bags under their eyes, and the sense of tension that follows them around. The thing that is so damaging about emotional stress is that eventually it turns into chemical and physical stress as well.

> Life is not what it's
> supposed to be.
> It is what it is.
> The way you cope with it is
> what makes the difference.

It All Adds Up

Over the years I have grown very accustomed to meeting new patients who seem to be baffled about why their health is as bad as it is. Doing what I do for a living and being an outsider looking in, it is obvious to me why their health is so poor. Stress is cumulative. In the process of doing a case history with a patient, I can clearly observe that different stressors started to mount one after another, eventually culminating in bad health.

Let me give you an example. A patient came to see me last year, a thirty-three-year-old male who had been diagnosed with fibromyalgia. He sat in my exam room like a zombie. He almost seemed mentally retarded in his inability to answer questions or to comprehend what I was asking him. As it turns out, there was nothing mentally wrong with him. He was, however, on so many medications that it should have been illegal for him to drive a car. I discovered that he was racing bicycles when he was about thirteen years old and had a crash. He hurt his back, but as most teenagers do, he just went about his life. That was a major *physical* stress. My x-ray examination revealed that he had hurt his spine back then but never had any treatment for it. By the time he was nineteen, he had intense backaches for which he began taking pain medication. That was a major *chemical* stress. He continued to take different drugs for pain, which led to side effects and more drugs. By the time he was twenty-three, he was diagnosed with fibromyalgia. Having been in pain for years due to physical stress, he became depressed. That was major *emotional* stress. His job was very physically demanding—more stress. He took more and more medication (nine prescriptions), which added more stress, and his home life and finances were a wreck.

By the time I met him, his life was a disaster, all because of cumulative stress. Do you see how that works? Let's rewind this story and see how it might have turned out if each stress had been approached in a correct and timely manner.

1. When he hurts himself on his bike at the age of thirteen, he gets the appropriate spinal care he needs to correct the problem. This would have prevented the backaches he was experiencing at the age of nineteen and taken care of the original problem, *physical stress.*

2. At nineteen years old, he does not need to begin taking pain medications. This would have taken care of the second problem, *chemical stress.*

3. By the time he reached the age of twenty-three, he wouldn't have been dealing with physical pain for ten years and most likely would not have become depressed. This would have taken care of the third problem, *emotional stress.*

Can you see how this chain of events created enough cumulative stress to totally derail this man's life and health? Can you also see that if the correct swift and decisive action had been taken to begin with he probably could have avoided his health crisis? He may have still ended up with a physically demanding job, but it would have been a lot easier to handle. Wouldn't it just make more sense to address each type of stress as it arises and do everything you can to avoid stress before it happens? Sure it does, and that's what we will talk about next.

Learning How to Manage Your Stress Effectively

Having been involved in the personal development arena for the last fifteen years, I have been to many great seminars and read hundreds of books. On more than one occasion I have heard writers or speakers say something to the effect of, "I'm going to show you how to eliminate your stress." Um, no, you're not. As long as breath is flowing through your lungs, you will have stress. Translation: there's always going be trouble. The key is to learn how to maintain a balanced life and manage your obstacles and challenges successfully.

To handle the different stresses and strains in your life, you must have an effective plan of attack for the three-headed monster. Remember, this thing is a beast, and you must guard against all three phases: physical, chemical, and emotional. In the previous chapters on detox and nutrition, I have already taught you how to handle chemical stress. Likewise, from the chapter on exercise and the upcoming chapter on the nervous system, you will have gained more than the lion's share of knowledge about physical stress. I am just going to give you a very short recap of those two subjects here and spend more time discussing emotional stress.

To better handle *physical stress*:

- Exercise daily

- Get proper amounts of sleep

- Be sure to sleep in a proper position

- Make sure your work station is ergonomically sound

- Participate in a posture enhancement program

- Get your spine adjusted

- Utilize proper lifting techniques when doing yard work, housework, heavy lifting, etc.

To better handle *chemical stress*:

- Use medication only when absolutely, positively necessary

- Eliminate junk food from your diet

- Stop smoking!!

- Begin consuming all-natural, organic food

- Use all-natural cosmetics and toiletries

- Decrease your alcohol consumption

- If using recreational drugs, stop!

- Use all-natural household cleaning supplies and detergents

- If applicable, get properly checked for biotoxins like mold and Lyme

Now I will spend some time on handling *emotional stress,* since it is not addressed at length anywhere else in this book. So many people have problems with this challenge. First of all, I believe it is paramount to understand that everyone has emotional stress and that it's okay. As a matter of fact, it is part of the human condition. To me, it is despicable how many people in our society are made to feel like something is wrong with them or they need to take psychotropic drugs if they have emotional stress. Guess what? Everybody does! I would say that there is probably something wrong with you if you don't have stress. That should be a relief.

Secondly, you really have to analyze why you're stressed and where your stress comes from. If we boil it down, we really are the creators of our own stress. Wouldn't you agree with that? How we choose to handle each situation that is presented to us will determine whether or not we become stressed out. Let me give you an example. You are driving through traffic, and someone cuts you off. You have two choices.

1. You can allow your blood pressure to rise, get all worked up, start cussing and flipping your finger at the person, steaming about how this person wronged you, and feel offended.

2. You can just realize that this person is a human being who makes mistakes, just like all of us, and let it go. The driver's action was probably unintentional and nothing personal. In a day from now you won't even remember it happened. Besides, chances are that you have accidentally cut people off in traffic before too. Are you perfect?

So you see that how you choose to process this event will largely determine whether or not you experience emotional stress from the situation. The reality is that we are faced with dozens of situations every day, and we always have a choice as to how we respond. For most people, that response is conditioned by having watched your parents while growing up. If your mother or father were quick-tempered people who frequently flew off the handle about minor things, you may be following in their footsteps. But it doesn't have to be that way. You have the choice to say, "No, I'm not going to be like that!" Don't just say, "Oh well, that's the way I am." That's what quitters do, and you are better than that. This may seem like a small thing, but choosing to be someone who handles events in your life with perspective and rational thinking could prevent you from ending up as someone who has hypertension or a heart attack.

Realizing that you are in control of your thoughts and your reactions to all that life brings you can be very freeing. It may take a lot of practice, but you can develop the mental muscle to focus on the empowering aspects of your life, not so much on the negatives.

When you boil it down, you'll understand that by only focusing on the negatives you will experience stress. Let me give you a little news flash: there will always be storms in your life. There are always going to be obstacles that you have to navigate through, and that's just the way it is. This is true for everyone. The people who can accept the storms and still focus on the positives are the ones who will lead happy lives. It is your choice—totally your choice. It is 100 percent, absolutely your choice whether to be stressed or to not be stressed.

Managing Your Expectations

At the core, the reason that people experience stress and unhappiness is because their current life conditions do not match up to their current life expectations. For example, you might say that you are unhappy because you think you should have more money. In other words, you don't have what you think you should have. Your circumstances don't match up with expectations. Or, you might say you are unhappy because you think you should be married with children and you aren't. Again, you don't have what you think you should have, so your circumstances don't match up with your expectations.

This is at the root of most unhappiness. So what does one do about it? Well, I'm not one for lowering expectations. I already feel that most people aren't thinking big enough about what they can accomplish in life. That said, you either need to make your life circumstances match up to your expectations, or change your expectations.

I vote for increasing your circumstances.

To make it even more applicable to this book, your current health circumstances may not match up to where you think your health should be. Well, the solution is the same. You either need to do everything in your absolute power to increase your health, or you must lower your expectations of where you think your health should be. The choice is yours, but I'd hope you wouldn't lower your expectations.

Tic Toc, Tic Toc

Without question, one of the key factors I observe in stressful people is poor time management. Time management happens to be something that I'm pretty good at. Allow me to explain how stress results from poor time management.

Let's say when you wake up you know that you have a dozen things on your to-do list for today. Well, first of all, congratulations for having a to-do list. You're ahead of the pack.

So you have a lot to accomplish and only a day to do so. While you may be a hard worker and someone who gets things done, if you don't have a good plan and a realistic perception about how long things will take to do, you will end up causing yourself stress each and every day. For this example, let's say you have to prepare some packages and take them to the post office, go to a dentist appointment at 9 am, go grocery shopping, work out, check your e-mails, pick up the dry cleaning, be at a job interview at 3:30 pm, and bring a dessert to a dinner club meeting at 6 pm.

If you just wake up having to conquer this list without timelines for when you will do each thing, there is no way you'll make it through your day without stress. You will be late for one or all of your appointments, you will be stressed out in traffic, and you will be angry with anyone or anything that slows down your progress, even though it's your fault that you didn't plan properly. What is not evident on the above list of things to do is how long it takes to drive from place to place, how long you will need to shower, how long it will take you to prepare your packages, and how long it will take you to prepare your dessert for dinner club. Will you need to iron your clothes? Will you need to make phone calls in response to your e-mails? You must consider these details and plan for them.

One of my first mentors had a saying that I still use to this day: "if you don't have a plan for your day, the universe will provide one for you." That is so true. When you don't properly plan, all hell will break loose. That's the day you'll get a flat tire, your dog will run out the door and escape when you're trying to leave, there will be an accident on the freeway that slows you down—on and on it goes. When you're not prepared, Murphy's Law will be in full force, and you'll be stressed out of your mind.

In order not to fall victim to this problem, you need to become efficient at managing your time. That may sound like I'm beating an old drum, but this is a small thing that can make a magnificent difference in your level of emotional stress.

I recommend that not only do you have a to-do list, but write it in chronological order of when you will accomplish each task. Take just a moment when writing your list to contemplate the variables, such as drive time, showering time, possible traffic and other delays. Will your days then always go perfectly? Heck, no! Mine sure don't. But having that list is like having a detailed map. It keeps you on track and focused. When you veer off course, you can always look back at your list and figure out what you need to do in order to get back on track.

Perhaps you're a stay-at-home mom. If you're thinking, "Well, I don't really need to do all that," I beg to differ! Being a stay-at-home parent is one of the most difficult jobs there is. Having a plan for your day will allow you to breathe easier and not feel overwhelmed by all the tasks you need to accomplish. This also holds true if you are currently unemployed. Having a plan for your day will keep you focused, inspired, and on track as you continue to search for gainful employment.

The Best Emotional Outlet

Now that you are managing your time, it is crucial that you give your mind a break. If you are reading this book right now and have been dealing with chronic health problems, I know that there is probably a full-out war going on inside your head every day of your life. "When will I get better?" "Will I ever get better?" "Will I find another job?" "Will my health get worse?" "Will I be able to support my kids?" "Will I ever be able to achieve my dream life?" "Do I even know what my dream life is?" "Why do I still feel guilty over things that happened years ago?" "Am I doing the right thing?" "Will my family be supportive of what I want to do?"

I know that questions like these are probably flying around in your head repeatedly, at light speed, each and every day of your life. It is exhausting. It is depressing. It is defeating. It is getting you nowhere. So stop the madness and give your mind a break.

I have been a very spiritual person my whole life, involved in different churches and copious amounts of self-study. I can't remember a day in my life when I haven't prayed at least once. My spiritual life was tremendously enhanced when I learned about the power of meditation. Before you go bonkers over hearing the word *meditation*, hear me out. For much of my life I thought that meditation was weird, dangerous, and, dare I say, evil. Well, like most stupid fears, my concerns were born purely out of ignorance. I didn't know anything about meditation, what the purpose was or how to do it.

The word *meditation* is mentioned in all religious texts, including the Bible. So no matter what background you come from, that should ease your fears. There are many different forms of meditation, and one can choose how he or she participates in it.

For the purposes of stress relief, I will teach you a very basic but powerful meditation technique. Doing this daily will leave you refreshed and more confident, focused, energetic, and creative. I have found that when I am on track with consistent meditation, my life seems to hit on all cylinders. I can say for certain that my life is much better when I am meditating on a daily basis. In addition to the benefits I just mentioned, creating this kind of mental break will allow the cells of your body to function at a higher level, which of course leads to faster healing. There are numerous medical studies, especially in the areas of hypertension and heart disease, which show the positive benefits of meditating.

A simple, stress-relieving meditation

I can walk you through this meditation technique in just a few short sentences. First, make sure you are in a quiet room with no distractions. Do not have a phone, fax machine, or anything that makes noise near by. You are trying to achieve silence. Next, sit in a very comfortable position in a chair or on the floor, whichever you choose. I prefer to sit in a nice, comfortable chair in a normal seated position. Begin the meditation by closing your eyes, relaxing your hands into your lap, and taking in a slow, deep breath through your nose. As you breathe in, try to picture your breath coming in through your nostrils and filling your lungs. Slowly exhale through your mouth and continue to visualize your breath leaving your body. The key is to try and focus on your breath. Ultimately, you would like to get to a point where there are no thoughts going through your mind. Nothing. Just pure silence. I will tell you that it is very challenging to do so. Your brain is a thought machine, constantly turning, working, and thinking. But the more you practice, the better you'll get. When a thought does pop into your head, don't get frustrated. Just say to that thought, "Thank you, I'll get back to you later," and go back to focusing on your breath. Continue breathing in through your nose and out through your mouth slowly while focusing on your breath. The goal should be to do this for twenty minutes per day. If necessary, start off with ten. I promise that if you do this on a regular basis, it will absolutely change your life. No exaggeration. Meditation will change your life.

Find Your Purpose

One of the more common emotional stressors is the feeling that you don't know your purpose in life. And let me tell you, it is very common! Join the club. Strong majorities of people are in your shoes. Think about how many college-educated people are working in well-paying jobs and still not living their dreams. I could teach an entire seminar on this topic. In the interest of time, let me say just a few things about this.

It doesn't matter how old you are or what your situation is, you can discover your purpose. The important point is to be constantly moving forward. You should be reading books, investigating—diligently trying to discover who you are and what you love. I personally believe that when you are trying to move forward through personal growth, your purpose will be revealed to you. The honest truth is that most people already know what their purpose is but are terrified to pursue it. Is this true for you?

Look at it this way. Julia Child did not become the great chef that we remember her as until she was in her fifties! Think about that. She discovered her talents in her forties and didn't really become the author/TV personality we knew her as until about the age of fifty. If you have a conversation about the all-time greatest chefs, she will undoubtedly be at the top of everyone's list. They even have a whole room at Le Cordon Bleu in Paris named after her. For the French to name a room after an American you know she had to be something! But her talents and purpose weren't discovered until her middle age.

What are you waiting for? Begin pursuing your dreams at once. When you do, you will undoubtedly be met with obstacles and challenges. Dreams don't come easy. You have to keep kicking and scratching until you get there. The beauty is that when you do start living your dreams, it will dramatically decrease your stress levels. After all, when you are doing what you love, how much stress could there be?

What About Therapy?

I am a big believer in therapy; however, it is great for some people and not so great for others. I believe that through self-discovery and reflection, people can usually figure themselves out, but some people have experienced such traumatic events in their life that they should seek out therapy.

The most important factor is to make sure you find a therapist whose style and personality you connect with. In the movie *Good Will Hunting,* Matt Damon plays a troubled young man who must go to therapy by order of the court. He totally wrecks every therapy session he attends and drives his therapists away, one after another, until he meets Robin Williams. The personality of Robin Williams and his style of therapy win Matt Damon over, and they end up developing a terrific relationship. Together they are even able to help Damon overcome his inner demons.

I highly recommend you find a therapist that you are comfortable with who is not just going to prescribe psychotropic drugs. This is really important. Some people need those drugs, but they are few and far between compared to how many people are actually taking them. It is an atrocity how many patients I see who are on antidepressant drugs just because they are going through challenges. Its just life, people!

I know some people really have a hard time dealing with situations and events that have occurred in their life. A death in the family, a messy divorce, child abuse: the list goes on. If you are carrying around baggage from emotional traumas like these, I urge you to take action to resolve them. It could be the difference between a life you wake up thrilled about every day and a life where you dread even waking up. That action may or may not involve a therapist. For many people, just attending an inspiring seminar or reading an amazing book can begin to totally change their lives.

Whether you are somebody who needs therapy or not, I recommend that everyone embark on a path of self-discovery and growth. It's very simple. Keep reading books like this. I highly recommend that you start with the classic book *Think and Grow Rich* by Napoleon Hill. That book changed the course of my life. I have read it at least six times and will continue to read it. It has nothing to do with money and everything to do with living the life you desire. After that, I recommend the book *The Power of Intention* by Dr. Wayne Dyer. As highly as I speak about Hill's book, I like this one even better. I have read *The Power of Intention* several times and continuously reference it. For me personally, it is the best book I have ever read. Last and certainly not least, you must read *Awaken the Giant Within* by Anthony Robbins. It will absolutely lift you to a place of aspiration that you never thought possible. After that, continue to choose books that appeal to you. Before you know it, you will be living a more fulfilled life.

One last note about therapy. If you have been seeing the same therapist for several years and are no further along in resolving your problems or increasing your level of contentment or happiness, it's time to move on. It may be that the style of therapy you are involved in isn't right for you. Keep trying.

Massage Therapy

I cannot have a chapter devoted to stress without mentioning the merits of massage therapy. I am of the firm belief that everyone should get a massage from a professional therapist at least once per month. The benefits are out of this world. Doing this regularly will tremendously reduce your stress and tension. As always, find a massage therapist you are comfortable with and go for it.

Be Free

By learning how to master your stress instead of letting your stress master you, you will truly free yourself. Just remember, as we go through life there will always be storms ... always. You can count on it. I'm not being negative; that's just the way it is. If you are serious about reclaiming your life and building optimal health, you must put the principles in this chapter into action. Remember, God doesn't deliver you through the storm; he delivers you in the storm.

Action Steps:

- Be sure to address all three kinds of stress: physical, chemical, and emotional

- Develop an effective time management program for your life

- Find time to pray and meditate daily

- Begin working on finding and fulfilling your purpose in life

- Embark on a path of self-discovery and personal growth

Chapter 10

The Master System

Your posture affects and moderates every physiological function from breathing to hormone production. Spinal pain, headache, mood, blood pressure, pulse, and lung capacity are among the functions most easily influenced by posture.

~Dr. Rene Caillet, AJPM

Sometimes when new patients come in to my office, I am faced with a big challenge: to undo a lifetime of societally conditioned beliefs about what a doctor does to bring about healing in the body. Most Americans have been brought up to believe that a doctor gives you medicine to help you get well. In my practice, my staff and I are faced with the daunting task of teaching people a new way. The beauty of it is that the lives of those who really "get it" will be changed forever.

One of the core fundamentals of what I teach is the need to have your central nervous system (CNS) functioning at its highest possible level. It only makes sense that if the CNS controls everything that happens in your body, you would want it to be as healthy as possible. Right? Good, I'm glad you agree. The typical view of what a chiropractor does is to work on the spine. Well, that's only part of the truth. What a chiropractor really does is work on the nervous system. The spine happens to be the vehicle by which we make that happen.

Unfortunately, the public in general really doesn't understand what chiropractic is, or the need for it. When I am in a public setting, such as a party or other gathering, and I am introduced as a chiropractor, to this day I will still occasionally meet someone who reacts by grabbing his lower back or his neck and say, "Ooh, ow, my back hurts!" And then he'll break out in laughter, amused by his own joke. The funny part is that when somebody acts that way, I respond by saying, "Wow, I'm glad I didn't say I was a gynecologist!"

The point is that we work with the spine to improve nervous system function. That's what it's all about. Many people say to me, "I've never needed a chiropractor before." In their mind, what they mean is that they have never had an injury that required chiropractic treatment to heal. The truth is that if you have a spine, you need a chiropractor. If you have teeth, you need a dentist, right? You don't go to the dentist only when your teeth hurt; you go to keep your teeth and gums healthy. Likewise, I get my spine adjusted every week to maintain a healthy functioning spine and nervous system. This is the same reason why many people bring their kids to get adjusted on a regular basis.

Everything we have discussed thus far has been designed to do one thing, to improve the function of your body. To help you achieve the most optimal levels of health, we must improve all of your bodily functions. As has been discussed in numerous areas throughout this book, in most cases taking drugs only serves to cover up symptoms and does not in fact improve bodily function in the least bit.

To have a discussion about function, we must discuss the very thing that controls every cell, structure, and function in your body: the central nervous system. You've heard of *Gray's Anatomy right? Gray's Anatomy, 29th edition*, states, "The central nervous system controls and coordinates all organs and structures of the human body." That must be a pretty important fact if *Gray's Anatomy* places it at the very beginning of the book. But if that's true, how come when your body begins to break down and you go to the doctor, he or she never examines your nervous system? I ask all of my new patients this question in the orientation class that I teach, and everyone agrees that they never get a nervous system exam.

In the Beginning …

Approximately eighteen days after you are conceived, the first part of your body that is formed is something called the neural tube. The neural tube becomes your brain and spinal cord, which makes up your central nervous system. Shortly after that, some little buds grow off of the spinal cord; those become your nerves. After the nerves are formed, little buds grow off the end of them, and those become your organs.

Brain, spinal cord, nerves, organs. The reason that it happens in that order is because your organs would have no idea how to function without the brain telling them what to do. This remains true for the rest of your life. From birth to burial, your body relies on your brain to tell it how to function. This is the reason why we have such great success with patients by using Brain-Based Therapy (BBT).

Maintaining an Optimally Functioning Nervous System

Let's talk about how your nerves run your entire body. First of all, that statement cannot be argued. Your nervous system does run your entire body. Since that is true, you need to do everything in your power to keep your nervous system healthy.

The obvious question is how do you do that. For a doctor like me, the answer is easy. However, the average person on the street is never taught this kind of information. You didn't learn it in elementary school health class. You didn't learn it in high school biology class, and you didn't even learn it if you took college courses in anatomy and physiology. You darn sure haven't ever heard it in your doctor's office.

In order to understand how to keep your nervous system functioning at its highest possible levels, let's define what I'm talking about. For our purposes, I'm referring to a healthy brain, spinal cord, and nerves. We keep those three things healthy through, fuel, activation, and posture.

The Nervous System Defined

Brain. It should go without saying that this is the most important organ in your body. It controls every single thing that you do, say, or think. When the brain is hitting on all cylinders, it can produce magic in your life. Your brain can help you create your wildest dreams and is responsible for all your bodily functions. When it's healthy, it will allow your entire body to function at its peak.

Many people are walking around with health problems that are totally related to poor brain function, but they are never even examined for this. Understand that when I say poor brain function, I'm not referring to sickness, disease, or pathology. I'm simply talking about neurology that is not firing the way it should, just as a weak, unconditioned muscle doesn't work as well as a strong, shapely muscle. As is the case with muscle, a poorly functioning brain is usually due to bad nutrition, toxicity exposure, and insufficient stimulation. These things can be corrected, and when they are, your overall sense of well-being will increase dramatically.

In chronic sickness and disease, a bad brain is always involved! Did you hear what I just said? In chronic sickness and disease, a bad brain is always involved! This means that the person with fibromyalgia, hypothyroidism, multiple sclerosis, and all of those weird, undiagnosed mystery conditions are all suffering from a sick brain. Sure, they have other problems as well, but the brain is a major player here. It reminds me of a quote by Dr. Daniel Amen, who is one of the premier brain doctors in the world.

151

Most people throughout the world care more about their faces, their boobs, their bellies, their butt, and their abs than they do their brains. But it is your brain that is the key to having the face, the breasts, the belly, the butt, the abs, and the overall health you have always wanted.

Dr. Daniel Amen, brain expert

Therefore, it is critical to find a practitioner who has an understanding of how to correct brain health. If you can't fix your brain, you can't fix your body. One of the coolest things that I experience in my practice is a patient's reaction when I do something that immediately changes the function of their brain and nervous system. For instance, in the course of examination, I could discover that a patient has a balance problem. I could then do some neurological rehabilitation exercises, then recheck the balance issue, and see an immediate change. It is incredible to see what the brain and body are capable of, and I feel privileged to be able to witness it in my practice.

This topic is so important that I can't do it justice in one short chapter. Everything else that happens in your body is interconnected with your brain. This is why it is so important to keep the rest of your body healthy. For example as your liver and gut begin to fail, your brain will die at a proportionate rate. If you are eating crappy food, taking all kinds of drugs, and living a toxic life, you are destroying your brain.

Most people are very fearful of developing dementia as they age. The earliest signs of dementia are poor short-term memory, difficulty learning new things, difficulty with directions, the need to write everything down so you don't forget, and constantly forgetting appointments and tasks. If you are experiencing these problems, you'd better act fast and start taking care of your brain and body.

By utilizing Brain Based Therapy (BBT), a practitioner can create immense changes in your brain function. It requires a specific course of care, complete with nutrition and neurological therapy. Once you undergo BBT, your brain will be healthier than it has been in ages and your sense of overall well being will soar! BBT is also a critical component to overcoming chronic sickness and autoimmunity. The best part about it is that Brain Based Therapy does not require drugs or surgery.

Spinal Cord. This is your lifeline. Your spinal cord is an extension of your brain that runs down your spine. I don't think it is by accident that God created our central nervous system to be completely encased in bone. It is just too important to not have the protection that bone provides. We all know the story of Christopher Reeve, the actor famous for starring in the movie *Superman*. In 1995, Reeve became paralyzed after a horseback riding accident. He was thrown from his horse and fractured his first and second cervical vertebrae. As a result, he became a quadriplegic. He couldn't move his arms or legs, and some organs required mechanical assistance for his survival, including his lungs. Think about that for a second. He didn't have a bacterial infection. He didn't have a virus. What he did have was an absence of nerve flow below his neck and as a result was virtually dead from the neck down.

People walk around with similar problems on a smaller scale every day. The person who is losing light touch sensation in their nerve pathways because of interference with the back half of the spinal cord and the person who has chronic pain due to the pain inhibiting pathways in the spinal cord are both suffering from a minor version of spinal cord damage. This type of damage can be the result of a vast array of minor or major traumas that have taken place over the course of a person's life, from something as simple as playing football or doing gymnastics as a child or something as traumatic as being in a car accident.

It is critical to have your spinal cord in good health and functioning properly.

Nerves. Your nerves are probably one of the most likely culprits in a good majority of musculoskeletal problems. If the spinal cord is an extension of your brain, then your nerves are an extension of your spinal cord. In essence, your entire nervous system is one big connection of wires.

It is quite common for a bone in your spine to become misaligned and put compressive force on a nerve. This is referred to as a subluxation. This "compressive force" is more commonly known as a "pinched nerve." Pinched nerves resulting from spinal subluxations can cause you a world of problems, and I'm not just referring to pain. It is extremely important to understand that nerves can be interfered with for a long period of time before they ever cause pain. Let's say that you have a subluxation at your first lumbar vertebrae, L1. The L1 nerve also gives function to your bladder. It is possible that nerve interference at L1 could cause you to urinate more frequently than normal. This could go on for a year or more before that pinched nerve at L1 starts to cause lower back and/or leg pain. In the meantime, most people will have been put on a medication to treat overactive bladder, which will start them down the path of side effects and ill health; the real problem was at the L1 nerve root. Wouldn't it make more sense to fix that?

Keeping the Nervous System Healthy

Fuel. Like the rest of the body, your nervous system requires proper nutrition to remain healthy. In functional neurology, we call this "fuel." In addition to eating a clean, healthy diet, it is also important to supplement with healthy fats like omega-3 fish oils. You have to shop carefully for these supplements. Most of the fish oil supplements that my patients bring in to me to check for quality are store-bought. I've said it before and I'll say it again—you cannot buy good quality supplements in a store. To find the best quality fish oil for you and your family, contact your local natural healthcare physician or visit my website.

In addition to supplementing with the appropriate fish oils, eating an all-natural, organic, healthy diet is the best way to ensure that your brain is getting the fuel that it needs to operate at optimal levels.

Functional medicine doctors realize the necessity of having balanced blood sugar to fuel your brain. When your blood sugar is on a constant rollercoaster ride, it drives your body crazy. Most people who are suffering from any type of chronic health problem have a blood sugar issue that needs to be dealt with. It is very easy to get blood sugar under control when you know what you are doing.

Activation. This term is used to describe healthy stimulation to the nerves, spinal cord, and various lobes of the brain. We accomplish that through neurological exercises and spinal adjustments.

For example, let's say that in the course of our examination, I discover that one of your main problems is that the left side of your cerebellum is not functioning properly. I could have you hold your left hand out to your left side and write the alphabet in the air while I have you doing certain eye exercises to stimulate the left side of your cerebellum simultaneously. Over a course of care and such rehabilitation, we can get your cerebellum firing the way that it should.

Likewise, I can focus my adjustment techniques on only one side of your spine, which will stimulate one side of your cerebellum, if that is what I'm trying to accomplish. This is known as unilateral adjusting and is an excellent source of activation for the brain.

I highly recommend that you visit the website www.lumosity.com and start doing some of the brain training on their website. These activities are not side specific like the ones I explained above, so anyone can do them. They will provide tremendous stimulation for your brain and will also help ward off dementia and other brain-related problems.

Getting your spine adjusted also improves immune system function. In fact, many parents bring their children in to get adjusted if they have a cold or runny nose just to activate the immune system. I truly believe that the fact that I have been getting my spine adjusted weekly for the last eighteen years is one of the reasons that I was not only able to live through the mold ordeal but also achieve a full recovery.

Posture. We have a saying in chiropractic that "Posture is the window to your spine." Well, it's also the window to your nervous system. The reality is that your spine is your posture. If you are hunched over, shifted over, or bent over or if your head sticks way out in front of you, it's because your spine is that way. Simply put, if your posture is bad, your health is deteriorating. Think about the healthiest people you know. If they are truly healthy, I can almost guarantee they have good posture. It is essential for a healthy life.

Conversely, poor posture can lead to a vast array of health problems. That isn't only my opinion or the opinion of chiropractors. Consider the quote that I opened this chapter with: *"Your posture affects and moderates every physiological function from breathing to hormone production. Spinal pain, headache, mood, blood pressure, pulse, and lung capacity are among the functions most easily influenced by posture."* That comes from Dr. Rene Caillet, a medical researcher at the University of Southern California. Dr. Caillet has conducted a wealth of research that proves how devastating poor posture and a bad spine can be to your overall health.

Frequently when I point out how bad a person's posture is during an analysis, she will say something like, "I always thought I had good posture. I stand up straight all the time." It is important to understand that standing up straight doesn't always equal good posture. We need to look at certain landmarks on the body and see how things line up. Most people don't have good posture.

Before getting into functional medicine, the focus of my practice was always spine and posture correction. And now, even though my focus has changed to taking care of chronically sick people with functional medicine techniques, I still utilize spine and posture correction as a key component to my care programs. Why? Because it is essential to human life, optimal health, and healing; how can I leave it out?

Maintaining healthy posture is a life-long commitment. I will always get my spine adjusted and employ postural exercises in my life. It is only through postural-based chiropractic care and posture-enhancing exercises that this can be achieved.

Working out with weights is certainly a great thing to do, but it won't fix bad posture. That being said, I still believe that you need to do weight training to keep your body and posture from further degeneration. Also, it is critical that you do core strengthening. Working on your core will help you to have a better posture, but it won't fix deeply entrenched spinal problems.

But Doc, How Did My Spine Get That Way?

That is a question that I frequently hear after I've shown x-rays to a patient whose spine is a disaster. My answer is always the same: "I don't know. I would need to have a videotape of your entire life to tell you what events caused this." However, I can tell you that subluxations in the spine occur as a result of many different things. Here is a short list.

- The birth process itself

- Falling down repeatedly when you are learning how to walk

- Falling off of couches, beds, and chairs as a child

- Playing sports

- Falling off bicycles

- Carrying heavy backpacks

- Car accidents (even fender-benders)

- Heavy lifting

- Excessive sitting

- Sleeping in bad positions

- Stress (physical, chemical, or emotional)

- Repetitive motion

- Sitting in front of a computer

- Gravity

As I said, this is a small list from the multitude of things that can create spine and nervous system distress. I don't prescribe to the theory that spinal misalignments are the cause of all health problems. I mean, look at my mold situation. Was I sick because my spine was out of alignment? No, my spine was in great alignment, but I was being viciously attacked by a deadly biotoxin. But it is absolutely incredible how many health problems resolve or decrease by improving your spinal health. I have witnessed it countless numbers of times over my career, and I am still sometimes amazed how much a person's health changes by working on the nervous system through spinal adjustments.

A few years ago, one of my patients approached me and asked if I thought that chiropractic would be able to help her young daughter, who was suffering from a kidney reflux problem. I had seen that scenario once before a few years earlier, and we had great success, so I felt strongly that we might be able to help. To be clear, I don't claim to treat kidney reflux problems, but when you allow the nervous system to heal, which is what chiropractic does, anything is possible. Little Anna had great results. Here is her story, written by her mother, Colleen.

By three or four months old, our daughter Anna had already had a couple of very high (105 degree), unexplained middle-of-the-night fevers. After the second one, the pediatrician took a urine sample and determined that Anna had a urinary tract infection (UTI). An appointment was booked for her to see a highly respected pediatric urologist at Children's Hospital to run tests for reflux, a common and serious problem in little girls. It would take several months before the urologist was able to see Anna.

In the meantime, I talked with Dr. Kuhn about Anna. I had been a patient for about a year and felt my overall health had improved, and I was interested to see if chiropractic could help our daughter. The following outlines the next several months:

In November 2007, Anna, just under a year old, started seeing Dr. Kuhn as a preventative measure. This was after the first UTI and prior to the official reflux diagnosis.

In January of 2008, we took Anna to Children's Hospital for an ultrasound and a Voiding Cystourethrogram (VCUG). Although prepared by the pediatrician for the procedure, I had no idea what it would be like to go through it with Anna. A VCUG is essentially an x-ray of the bladder. In order to get a good picture, the patient needs to be perfectly still. The radiologist inserts dyed liquid and inflates the bladder. The patient cannot move, and the procedure is not complete until she has voided the liquid from the bladder. This meant that Anna, at that time under a year old, was strapped to a table while they inserted a tube into her urethra, filled her bladder, and held her down until she peed while they took x-rays. There is not much that is more difficult than watching your child hurt and afraid. Anna was diagnosed with kidney reflux on both sides. Her kidneys were undersized, and the reflux was a grade III/IV (on a scale of I to V, with V being the highest damage).

In January 2008, Anna had her first official exam with Dr. Kuhn. He began adjusting her weekly, and she has had continued adjustments since then.

The plan from the urologist indicated that every time Anna had a fever over 100 degrees with no other medical signs (i.e., ear infection, positive strep, etc.) she would be catheterized to check for the presence of a UTI. Although the catheterizations are difficult, painful, and potentially traumatic for the child, the theory is that an infection in a child with kidney reflux can quickly scar and damage the kidneys. Therefore, the problem needs to be addressed immediately. Anna was catheterized during multiple visits following low-grade fevers. All were negative for a UTI. With the pediatrician, we then decided that Anna would not be catheterized unless a fever was higher than 103 degrees. Although the pediatrician had her standard protocol she was supportive and responsive to my research, willing to listen and to treat Anna in a way that I was comfortable with.

The initial protocol from the urologist included starting Anna on a low dose of daily antibiotics (Bactrim). It was expected that she would stay on them until she was five years old. In theory, this would either keep the UTIs from forming at all or stop the infection from scarring her kidneys.

After a few months, the pediatrician sent Anna back to the urologist for a routine ultrasound. The news was certainly not as good as we had hoped. Anna's kidneys were not growing; in fact, they appeared even smaller, and there was a concern that they were shrinking.

I continued to discuss our concerns about daily antibiotic use with the doctors and agreed to try the protocol and proceed accordingly. They expected Anna would be on the Bactrim until the reflux was resolved or she had surgery. I decided after eight months with no further incidents to wean her off the antibiotics.

Through all of this Anna continued to see Dr. Kuhn. Anna loved going to see him and getting adjusted. She understood that it was helping make her healthy. Every time we put her up on the table at the pediatrician's office she would cry; however, she would excitedly run into Dr. Kuhn's office every week!

Just after Anna's second birthday we took her back to Children's Hospital for the follow-up VCUG. Her nana came with us, prepared with a talking teddy bear, lots of love, and a tea party to help Anna pee quickly. By this time Anna was old enough to be afraid of the procedure, regardless of how kind the staff was. She was amazing ... scared and upset but not hysterical. She peed quickly, and the painful, invasive procedure was over relatively quickly (fifteen minutes instead of the previous thirty minutes).

We waited patiently for the urologist to come and see us with her results. I was prepared with research and information indicating why the Bactrim wasn't working and why we shouldn't proceed with the prescribed surgery at age four or five if the reflux did not resolve. The urologist couldn't hide her shock when she walked through the door; I almost passed out. I thought for sure something was really bad. She flipped open the chart and told us that she was just going to get right to it. She said she had never seen anything like this. Then she said it was gone, all of it, gone. There was no reflux, no sign of the reflux, no scarring. In the best-case scenario, they would usually hope that the kidneys had grown a bit and they could downgrade her to a lower number. She said at this point she wouldn't even categorize Anna as having reflux … at all.

According to common research, spontaneous resolution is progressively less common in grades III and IV (only about 10 percent of grade IV involving both sides), and rare in grade V. Anna was an anomaly. The pediatric urologist told us she literally did not need to see us again, ever. Unless Anna had a repeat UTI, she did not need any follow-up. I sat there in tears. We were stunned.

At five years old, Anna now says that God and Dr. Rob made her healthy. She knows how much we prayed for her, and she knows that Dr. Rob helped. Nana and I say that God healed her but he used Dr. Kuhn's hands. She is now a happy, healthy five-year-old with no lasting effects from the reflux. Dr. Kuhn still regularly adjusts her.

I would like to say that Anna's story was a miracle, but miracles are things that don't happen very often. We regularly see patients getting their lives back with the work that we do and yes, sometimes it does seem miraculous. I mean, think about it. This little girl had a problem with her kidneys and all we did was influence her nervous system with simple little adjustments to her spine and it changed her life. I feel very blessed to have been a helping hand to this beautiful child.

What's The Big Deal About Posture?

Why would bad posture affect your health? Consider this research by Dr. Alfred Breig, a prominent German neurosurgeon. When somebody displays a posture where the head sticks forward, it is known as Forward Head Syndrome (FHS). In most cases the person has lost the natural cervical curve in their neck. This is what Dr. Brieg's research revealed: "Loss of the cervical (neck) curve, the arc of life, stretches the spinal cord five to seven centimeters and produces pathological tension, putting the body in a state of disease."

I have seen cadaver studies that involve cutting the spine in half, and the findings are stunning. In cadavers with a normal curve in the neck, the spinal cord is relaxed, the discs are normal, and there is an absence of arthritis. On the flip side, in cadavers without the cervical curve, the spinal cord is pulled taut, the bottom of the brain stem is pulled on, and there is disc degeneration and spinal arthritis. This is the pathological tension and state of disease that Dr. Brieg is referring to.

The challenge with these types of problems is that they are very insidious in nature, which means that they creep up slowly. In many instances they do not produce symptoms, even though they are creating sickness, disease, and a lowered state of health in the body. I've lost track of the number of patients over the years that have been able to throw away useless medications once we began correcting their nervous system.

This is why it is so critical to maintain a healthy posture. Your spine is your posture, and your nervous system's health depends on it.

> Look well to the spine for
> the cause of disease.
> ~Hippocrates

How Does This Apply to You?

You began reading this book to either find out how you can overcome a chronic health problem or to take your already good health to the next level. So what do you do with what you learned in this chapter? Even though I did not write this book with the intention of trying to turn people on to chiropractic, I know without a shadow of a doubt that it is a key component to living a healthy life.

As I stated earlier, I have been getting my spine adjusted on a regular basis for eighteen years. I don't do it because I have spinal problems, because I don't. I do it to maintain health, and I suggest that you and your family do the same. There are numerous techniques and philosophies within the chiropractic profession. I suggest you find one that suits you best and that you are comfortable with.

If you are suffering from any type of chronic pain syndrome, autoimmunity or some other mystery condition, chiropractic adjustments might not be enough. You will probably need some neurologic work and help with cleaning up your metabolic system. However, some of the best functional medicine doctors in the world are chiropractors, and if you find the right one it will change your life.

If you already see a doctor of chiropractic and you are happy, stick with it and make it a regular thing. Finding the right doctor for you can be tricky. Go to my website and click on the "find a doctor" section, and I will help lead you in the right direction. You should know that whomever I refer you to will be somebody very versed in functional medicine and could be the right person to lead you back to health.

Action Steps:

- Be sure to eat an all-natural, healthy, organic diet and supplement with omega-3 fish oil for optimal brain nutrition.

- Begin a weight-lifting program and incorporate core-strengthening exercises to help improve your posture.

- Become aware of your posture when you stand or sit. If you are slouching, stand or sit up straighter. This won't fix a bad spine, but it will slow down the degenerative process.

- Find a chiropractor and set out on a lifetime course of spine and nervous system health.

Chapter 11

The Healing Power of Belief

When you believe passionately in that which
does not exist, you create it.

~Nikos Kazantzakis (paraphrase)

The first time I encountered the above quote was while reading the book *Being in Balance*, by Wayne Dyer. If you've never read it, I highly recommend it. I would like you to think deeply about what that sentence actually means. Kazantzakis, a Greek writer and philosopher, is telling us that our beliefs create our life. Anyone who has studied self-improvement or personal development knows this to be a universal truth. However, the majority of people inhabiting our planet, even educated ones, are either not in tune with this knowledge, don't believe it, or look down upon it as "voodoo."

My life's work, my self-study, and my own spiritual journey have taught me the power of belief. I know full well that the reason I have had so much success in my life is due to a never-ending belief in my ability to accomplish what I set out to do. Likewise, I know the reason that I was able to recover from the mold sickness is because no matter how bleak things seemed, I never relinquished my belief that I would find health again.

I know that in this book I have taught you the true path to healing and given you cutting-edge information. I have opened your eyes to ugly truths and revealed things that you don't normally hear in a doctor's office. It is my firm belief that if you do the things I have taught you, your health will improve dramatically and you will have the best chance of overcoming sickness. However, if you don't truly believe that you can be healthy again, it is all for naught.

This is consistent with every spiritual background. All spiritual texts talk about the power of believing in yourself, in what you are doing, in what you are praying for, etc. In the New Testament, Jesus states: if you *believe*, you will receive whatever you ask for in prayer. (Matthew 21:22) The operative word in that phrase is believe. I think due to our humanness, we often times minimize the importance of these words when we should be maximizing them. There are numerous other such statements in the Bible and all other religious documents discussing the power of belief.

An overwhelming majority of people in the world claim to have belief in a higher power. It doesn't matter what your background is. Since all religious texts tell us about the power of belief, don't you think we should listen? By no means am I trying to turn this into a religious debate. I just want you to really grasp the importance of having belief in yourself and your abilities.

Is There Really a Link Between Positive Thinking and Good Health?

You better believe there is. The amount of research done and anecdotal evidence out there to back this up is staggering. Not only does positive thinking link with good health, negative thinking links with bad health. In the smash hit bestselling book *The Power of Positive Thinking* by Norman Vincent Peale, Peale quotes Dr. Dunbar: "It is not a question of whether an illness is physical or emotional, but how much of each."

Dr. Dunbar is saying that there lies within the cause of every illness a component of emotional distress. I'm not suggesting that if you are suffering from fibromyalgia or ulcerative colitis that it's because you are a negative thinker, although if you are a negative thinker, it is certainly making you worse. What I am suggesting is that if you doubt the fact that you can ever overcome your illness, you surely never will.

What do you believe about your health? What do you believe about your chances for a full recovery from whatever ails you? What do you believe about your ability to achieve the highest levels of optimal health? Positive answers to these questions will be a major plus to your future health, while negative answers will be a catastrophic detriment.

When you think positively about your body and your health, chemical reactions take place at the cellular level that improve all of your bodily functions. Think about that. Thinking positively in regards to how you see your health and what you can accomplish in terms of healing actually makes you healthier! Does that mean that if you are in the middle of a major sickness or chronic pain flare-up that thinking positively will suddenly make it go away? Maybe not. But if you are in the middle of that same situation and all you can think about is how miserable you are and that you will never get well, you will definitely slow the process down. So stop it! Negative thoughts about your health also create reactions in your body at the cellular level, and of course, those reactions are damaging and will help to ensure that you remain in a poor state of health.

Having been at a point where I literally thought that I would die, I know full well what it means to feel like there is no hope. It is at those lowest moments, where things seem the bleakest, that you must fight to truly believe in your recovery. During the time that your body is the sickest and most inflamed, your cells are looking for all the help they can get.

High Frequency/Low Frequency

Every cell in your body has a frequency. Yes, the body truly is electric. The faster the frequency, the healthier the cell is. Slower frequencies push the cells toward a lowered state of health. The brain exudes a tremendous amount of influence over cellular frequencies. So here's where your thoughts come into the picture.

Positive thoughts are high-frequency thoughts. When you think positively, you increase the frequencies of every cell in your body. This literally means that when you are a consistently positive thinker, you increase the health of all the cells in your body.

Conversely, negative thoughts are low-frequency thoughts. When you think negatively, you decrease the frequencies of every cell in your body. This literally means that when you are a consistently negative thinker, you decrease the health of all the cells in your body.

I want you to stop for a moment and really consider the implications of what this all means. Your thoughts literally have the ability to make you healthy, or they can make you seriously sick. You have to choose what level of health at which you really want to live. It has not been predetermined for you by your genetic code! I'll speak more on genetics in just a moment, but you *must* realize that you can live at the level of health that you want to live. Believe me, I know first-hand that it can be very challenging to keep up a positive outlook when you are going through a long-term health crisis, but you must do so. It is critical. If you are already enjoying a life of good health, you must still keep a positive outlook on your health to fend off experiences you will encounter as you age.

Negative thinking was a big reason why my mother died at the age of sixty-three. As far back as I can remember, my mom viewed herself as a sick person. She was a hypochondriac for sure; she always thought something was wrong with her, even when there wasn't. When I would tell her to exercise, there was always an excuse for why she couldn't do it. When I attempted to counsel her on better eating habits, another excuse came. I can remember her taking medications, both over-the-counter and prescriptions, every single day of her life. It's no wonder her health deteriorated so badly at the end of her life. The funny thing is, she was never really sick. There was never anything wrong with her, yet she took meds every day and went to the doctor all the time! She always talked about having a bad heart, but there wasn't anything wrong with her. Guess what she developed at the end. That's right, a weak heart. Her negative thoughts turned out to be a self-fulfilling prophecy, and they destroyed her life.

To mirror that story, I have always been a positive thinker. The last several years have presented more than enough opportunities for me to abandon my optimism, but I won't. There were days back in 2007 and 2008 when I was so sick that I thought for sure I was going to die soon. I had to stop myself and turn that thought process around. I constantly prayed, meditated, and visualized myself returning to good health. In the end, I did. That is the power of positive thinking.

Genetics, Schmenetics!

Far too many times I have seen beliefs about genetics or family history completely derail somebody's life. Over the years I have frequently heard comments like "Well, my dad had heart disease, so I know that I will too." Or, "My mom had cancer, so I know that I probably will too." Are you really going to let family history determine the course of your life? If I lived my life according to that line of thinking, I guess I'd be lucky to make it to sixty-five, since both of my parents died early. Guess what? I'm still planning on living to a hundred!

So what is the deal with genetics? How much do they really affect your life and your future? Look at it this way. I've read many times before from different sources that only 5 percent of all cancers are genetic. Do you understand how absolutely huge that last statement is? This means that 95 percent of all cancers that are destroying people's lives are caused by the environments to which we expose ourselves. Toxicity, poor food choices, smoking, alcohol, stress, excessive medicating, and numerous other factors are responsible for causing all these cancers and other health problems.

In Bruce Lipton's book *The Biology of Belief*, he brilliantly describes what I am talking about. The reality is that epigenetics are far more important than genetics. Epigenetics refers to how internal and external environmental factors regulate gene activity. Lipton explains that your genes are constantly being remodeled and reshaped in response to environmental factors and your beliefs about your body. So your genetics don't have nearly as much impact on your health as what you do to yourself does.

Once again, do you understand the enormity of that? This means that the things you do and believe will determine how your health unfolds! It also means that if you are willing to change how you treat your body and what you believe about your ability to be healthy, you can literally mold your physical health into whatever you want it to be. In Lipton's book, he wonderfully explains this process, complete with all the cellular research to back it up. I strongly recommend that you read *The Biology of Belief.* There is much more to it than this two-paragraph recap here.

The bottom line is that it's time you started believing in your health and your future. If you don't, you'll never reach the level of health that you want. More importantly, quit believing in that stupid, old, outdated philosophy that you are doomed by your parent's blueprint.

> Those who are willing to spend a few years doing what most won't, can spend the rest of their lives doing what most can't.

A Self-Fulfilling Prophecy

Earlier, when I was talking about my mother's negative belief system, I mentioned that she had a self-fulfilling prophecy. Do you know what that term means? It has become quite popular over the last decade, and I want to talk about it a little. A big part of what I do is inspire people not only toward better health but a better life. I am a big-time dreamer and not ashamed to admit it. If we only go around once, we'd better grab all we can and have as many breathtaking experiences as possible. That's the way I see it.

My wife and I have had numerous talks together over the years about this very topic. Sometimes when life is kicking your ass, it's important to stop and remind yourself of the mission that you are on. Wendy and I have had to do that for each other numerous times when going through stressful situations. As I near the completion of this book, we recently had another of these talks, specifically discussing how we want this book to affect the world and how we can further inspire people to live better lives.

Just about everyone at one time or another has experienced a self-fulfilling prophecy, but probably few have realized that they did so. A self-fulfilling prophecy is when you constantly think, talk, act, and believe in a certain way, which eventually becomes your reality. Let me give you an example.

A young family used to come to my practice in Phoenix a number of years ago. The husband and wife were just about my age then, and they had three young children. I really liked them a lot, and they were loyal to my practice. There was one very striking characteristic about them as a family: they were the most negative people I had ever met. Negativity just dripped off of them like bad cologne. Every other phrase out of their mouths was something negative about their life or circumstances. You would constantly hear phrases like, "Well, with our luck ..." or "That's just our luck, you know ..." or "It probably won't work out." The self-pity was mortifying, and the lack of expectations for anything good was unbelievable.

This family's negativity was a never-ending self-fulfilling prophecy. Not surprising to me, this is a list of all the bad things that happened to them in just the few years that I knew them:

- The father had two pretty serious injuries
- The mother and kids were involved in a horrific car accident
- The father lost his job
- They went bankrupt
- Her parents had several serious health problems
- His parents were killed in a car accident

They expected the worst, and life gave it to them. They were always speaking negatively about what they expected to happen to them, and life didn't disappoint them. Do you do this? You had better examine this question seriously. I see it every day. I would say that, generally speaking, majorities of people are negative. Patients come in all the time saying things like, "There is a virus going around work, so I'm sure I'll get it." Oy! You cannot afford to think that way! What you should be thinking is, "Everyone at work is getting sick, but it's not going to get me."

The Law of Attraction

The phrase *law of attraction* has become pretty prominent since the release of the book *The Secret* in 2006. *The Secret* was put together by author Rhonda Byrne and contains many contributions by other authors: doctors, success coaches, and leaders in quantum physics. To be clear, *The Secret* is an oversimplified version of how the law of attraction works, but it gets the fundamental point across. The basic idea is that whatever you think about shows up in your life. Be careful. Many people take that as an excuse to not take action. No, it's not just as simple as thinking "I want a million dollars," and it shows up. There is much more to it than that. Positive thinking without massive action is a complete waste of time.

I did enjoy *The Secret*, but I know for a fact that nothing comes to fruition without massive action. I'm in total agreement with Tony Robbins on this subject. You must take action. However, I do believe that the law of attraction is working in all of our lives, and it is really important to understand it. Personally, my favorite book on the law of attraction is *The Power of Intention* by Wayne Dyer, which I have already mentioned. The point is that these books can really teach us a lot about how our beliefs affect our health and our lives.

Let me give you the basics. Please do not let your religious beliefs or any lines of societal conditioning throw you off here. Just take it for what it is. Think of yourself as a cell phone tower. You are constantly sending out messages into the universe, and you, the tower, are constantly receiving messages from the universe. Those messages vary in frequency, and like attracts like. If your tower is sending out low-frequency messages (negative), it will be receiving low-frequency messages. If it is sending out high-frequency messages (positive), it will be receiving high-frequency messages. Pretty easy to follow so far, right?

Well, let's say that your tower is constantly sending out messages that you are afraid you will get sick and that you are tired of always being sick. Guess what is coming back to you? More sickness. On the flip side, if you are sending out messages that you are healthy and that you feel so blessed to be enjoying good health, guess what is coming back to you? More health! That may sound ridiculous, but it's true. Just remember, you still have to act on your thoughts. Action is the key. Whether positive or negative, the more action you take, the stronger those frequencies will get. So, if you are negative and you consistently take action toward being negative, or you exhibit inaction, you will get more of the negative. If you are positive and you take massive, positive action, you will receive more positives.

I want to stress that there is a tremendous amount of research out there to back up what I am saying. I highly encourage you to study quantum physics. Albert Einstein was one of the first to discuss quantum theory, which basically explains how everything in the universe vibrates at certain frequencies. I have read about devices that can actually measure the frequency of your thoughts and how those thoughts affect your health. The point is that we are like antennas that attract into our lives exactly what we put out.

The negative family members that I spoke about earlier had a black cloud hanging over their heads. No matter where they went or what they did, something bad would happen to them. It was like the worst catch-22 you could imagine. They are negative people, so they attract negative circumstances into their lives. Those negative circumstances then reinforce the negative thoughts and feelings that they constantly experience, so the wheel just goes around and around: a self-perpetuating machine.

Am I saying that bad things never happen to positive people? No way. Not in the least. Look at what happened to my family. We are very positive people, and we had a run of bad things happen to us, starting with the mold exposure, which was unprecedented in my life. In the beginning, I had no idea why those things happened to us. Now I know that it was brought to us to make me a stronger leader and make us a stronger family. I can tell you that when the whole mold thing started I was at a point in my life when I was more committed to church, my relationship with God, my tithing habits, self-study, prayer, meditation—everything. From an analytical standpoint, I cannot come up with one reason why it should have happened, but it did. You know what? That's life. Bad things do happen to good people sometimes.

I can tell you this. Due to my sickness, lowered productivity at work, and the resulting stress in my relationships, I do believe the overall lower energy that I was temporarily living with definitely slowed down my return to good health and prosperity. Am I saying that I was being negative? Yeah, a little. And even when I was being positive I wasn't living at the same high level of energy that I was used to. I don't beat myself up over it. It's part of being human.

What I want you to realize about the law of attraction is that it is real, and it is working in your life, either for you or against you. Whether it works for or against you will be determined by the thoughts, beliefs, and actions that you display every day of your life.

Using Your Beliefs to Create Better Health

You can see how important it is to adopt better beliefs about what is possible for you and your health. One thing I can't stand is when doctors tell people, "You will just have to learn to live with it." That's the best they can do?

You don't have to learn to live with it; you need to learn to get past it. It starts with the belief that you cannot only be well, but that you can live at an optimal level of health. Remember, no matter where you are at in your walk with health or what ails you, someone else has had it worse and made a comeback. Never forget that! I know people will accuse me of giving false hope to very ill people, but I believe that as long as you have a breath in you, there is room for a miracle. Will every cancer patient make a full recovery? Of course not, but if they don't believe they have a chance, then they are finished before they get started.

Start today. First, just decide that you believe amazing things are possible for your body and your health. Truly make that decision now. This is the first step. It's not enough just to say that you'll start being more positive. You must really believe that good health is possible for you.

Now that you've decided that good health is possible for you, you must also decide that you will achieve it. As nice as this all sounds, good health won't show up on your doorstep just because you decide to think more positively. You have to want it, badly! You have to commit to achieving it. You have to say to yourself, "Okay, I'm going to regain my health, and I'm absolutely not going to stop until I get there!" Once you've done that you are on your way.

Next, start to visualize living at the level of health that you want or overcoming XYZ condition. You need to set aside some time to just sit quietly, uninterrupted, every day and visualize yourself being healthy. Close your eyes and see yourself as that person you envisioned in chapter 4 when we created the new you. See yourself waking up every day with abundant energy and no pain. See yourself eating healthy and not taking any medications. See yourself fifty pounds lighter if you need to lose weight. See yourself running in a 10K race if that is appropriate for you. You get the picture. Visualize these things and believe them. Feel them. Love them and own them.

Lastly, participate in whatever spiritual habits you utilize in your life in reference to good health. In other words, if you like prayer, pray for your health. Pray with feelings of expectation and hope for a better life. Do not pray from desperation and despair. That is almost as bad as negative thinking. Don't do it. If you like to meditate, meditate on good health, healing, and expectations for a fantastic life. Again, see it all from the positive.

Your beliefs about your health will have more of an impact on your physical body than just about any habit you can have. If you truly adopt a positive belief system about what is possible for your health, you will be unstoppable. You will find that you can quit smoking or lose weight effortlessly. Things that used to seem hard will quickly seem easy. Think positively about your health each day, and soon you will find yourself building healthy habits like eating good food and exercising. As a benefit, you will notice that you have better energy, more joy, and higher expectations. Don't you deserve that?

Remember, "When you believe passionately in that which does not exist, you create it." Believe passionately in your good health, and start creating it today!

Action Steps

- Realize that your thoughts create frequencies, which can affect the level of health in your cells. Begin to develop positive thinking habits today

- Read the book *Biology of Belief* by Bruce Lipton

- Understand that the law of attraction is working in your life, but you must take intentional action towards creating better health

- Make the decision that you will live at the highest level of health possible

- Pray, meditate, and visualize your best health every day

Chapter 12

It's Time to Take Back Your Life!

Fall down seven times, stand up eight.

—Japanese proverb

Pick up a magazine or turn on the television and you will find them: true stories of people who overcame the odds, who were told they only had a short time to live and now are in perfect health. Some were literally on their deathbeds, and they not only survived but came back to live extraordinary lives. If they can, you can too! You can get your life back; you can return to health, and you can live the life of your dreams!

Living with chronically poor health can certainly knock you down. It can knock you out. Let's be honest, it can knock the living shit out of you. I know—it did to me. In my eyes, getting better just wasn't good enough. I wanted my life back. I had spent an entire life respecting my body and my health, and, doggone it, I wanted them back! My comeback was slow: methodical, steady, and filled with plenty of ups and downs. Just when I'd think I was doing well, I'd experience a full-on relapse of mold symptoms. Round and round the rollercoaster went.

How was I able to do it? That's very easy. If you've made it this far in the book, then you already know. I utilized all the principles that I've taught you in these pages. I properly detoxed my body of the mold and repaired my gut and liver. My already-good diet got a heck of a lot better in a hurry! I exercised whenever I could and made sure that I was getting enough rest. I prayed and meditated like nobody's business and continued to receive spinal adjustments. Most importantly, I held the firm vision and belief in my mind's eye that I would regain my health. Remember, it wasn't just me going through this episode; my entire family participated in all of the things I just mentioned. Even my youngest son, who was only five years old at the time, went through this process.

I now know that my family had to endure this experience so that I could better understand chronically ill people and walk the path of functional medicine. In the few years since I was sick, the extent to which I've been able to help patients is exponentially greater than before. The learning experience that resulted from going through that whole mold situation brought me to this level and this point in my life.

Does everything always come up roses? Of course not. Any mature, reasonable person knows that. Your life is not supposed to be perfect. If you're taking antidepressants because your life isn't perfect, guess what? It's not supposed to be! Don't go along with the masses and put your body through a toxic chemical hell like the rest of America is. Dare to be different. Take care of your body. Figure out the hidden causes of your chronic problems and work toward fixing them. Your life will only get better if you do.

I can hear the naysayers now: *"Oh, Dr. Rob, you don't understand my situation ..."* Blah, blah, blah. Listen, I don't want to be harsh here, but I care about you, so I want to tell you the truth that maybe nobody else will. No matter where you are at, somebody else has had it worse than you and made a comeback. Enough said.

My fourteen-year-old son Nick saw a motivational speaker today as part of a school field trip. The man was born without arms or legs. This guy is successful, and he's happy! Why do you think that is? Because he made the choice that he wasn't going to let life's circumstances get him down. You think you have problems? Look at him.

You might respond, "Well, yes, Dr. Rob, but I am dying. I have XYZ condition, and I've only got a few months to live." My honest, sincere heartfelt reply to you would be, "I am so sad to hear of the predicament that you are in. Truly. Remember, no matter what's going on with you, someone else has made a comeback from it. If I can lead you to the right answers that help you become the next great comeback, let me know. I'll do everything I can, because, friend, that's what I am here for. If you choose to go quietly into the night, I will absolutely respect that decision, but I hope you'll give life one more try."

I love life. I plan on living a long, fulfilling life. You only go around once, so you have to make it the best damn life you can! I want to see the world. I want to see my kids succeed. I want to meet my grandkids and see them grow up. I want to help lead as many other people to health, happiness and success as I can. I want it all, and I'm not afraid to say that. No apologies here. I hope you'll adopt the same attitude. You deserve it! You deserve to be happy, you deserve to be healthy, you deserve to be successful, and you deserve to have it all!

Again? Really?

On Monday, November 7, 2011, while I was about halfway through writing this book I had an experience that you won't believe. It was a pretty cold day, the first day of the winter I needed to turn the heater on in my office. I turned on the heat in the treatment area and then went back to my private office for a few minutes.

Upon returning to the treatment area I immediately encountered an awful musty smell and noticed a few little white flakes coming out of one of the air vents. I immediately shut the heater off and told Rebecca, my assistant, to call an A/C guy and have him come check it out. The next day the A/C guy came out and started inspecting the units. I was in my office when Rebecca walked in and said, "You better come hear this for yourself." Uh oh!

The A/C guy proceeded to tell me that the drainage lines from the unit had a problem and that there was a massive amount of mold in my office. *What the hell?* was literally the first thing that went through my mind, followed by, "You've got to be freaking kidding me!" Of all things that I could be exposed to, nothing is worse than mold! My body is highly sensitive to it, and I could easily relapse into symptoms. This was a *major* problem

This is why I chose the quote that opens this chapter. You fall down seven times, stand up eight. That's all there is to it. Life is going to throw you some curve balls. You either deal with them and learn how to hit the curve ball or you strike out. Which are you going to choose? I chose to fight this menace again. I used my belief system I discussed in chapter 11 to the best of my ability. I firmly believed that no matter what happened, that mold was not going to effect me. Well, you know what? It did, a little, but for the most part I came out okay. I had a few symptoms here and there, but not too bad overall. I chose health! I chose life! And so should you.

You miss 100 percent of the shots that you never take!

Choosing a Better Life

In this book I have shown you how to create better health and therefore a better life. Your health is the foundation of everything you do. Without it, things seem bleak; with it, you feel unstoppable. It is my greatest hope that reading this book will push you to choose a better life.

It really is a choice. No matter how good or how positive you are, it's easy to let life knock you down. Wendy and I had a great discussion recently; we both recognized that the circumstances of our life had really beaten us down a few notches. The first thing to realize is you still have to take responsibility. Yes, it's true that we had some really bad things happen to us, but it is our job to maintain the same level of belief that we always had. We didn't do that for a while, and it took quite some time for us to recognize it.

We are the kind of people who always keep moving forward. We work hard, we have vision, and we believe that the outcome will be in our favor. Because of that, it was hard for us to see that our level of positivity and belief in ourselves had faded a bit. Most people wouldn't have noticed. We set high standards for ourselves and were still raising our kids, living our lives, and leading the way business as usual. However, when the smoke cleared and we really stopped to analyze where we were at, it was crystal clear to Wendy and I that we had sunk down quite a bit. Instantly, we made the choice that we would turn that around, and we have, in a major way.

Now it's your turn. I want you to decide right now that you will live a better life. No matter what your circumstances are, I want you to decide that you will improve, that you will turn your life around, and that you will regain your health. If you are already healthy, I want you to commit to taking it to the next level so that you can live an incredibly long, happy life.

Making that decision is the first critical component to success. Once you have done that, you must decide that you will not stop until you get there, period! Nothing is going to get in your way. Go back to chapter 4 and reread the part about creating the vision of the new you. Repeat that drill several times if you must, until you have a firmly held vision of what you want your health, your body, and your life to look like. The rest is gravy.

All you have to do now is begin implementing the steps I taught you in this book. If you will require functional medicine testing to figure out why you have a chronic problem, begin your quest at once to find a functional medicine doctor. If you know of someone in your area, go see him or her. Ask around. Do some research. Should you not find anyone, go to my website and ask me or look on our resource page to find a doctor. You can't afford to wait. You've been dealing with poor health for long enough. The time to take charge is now.

Commit to adopting the concepts I've taught you about detoxification, healthy eating, exercising, proper sleep habits, stress reduction, and positive thinking. If you do, your life will change dramatically in a short period of time.

I'm not afraid to tell you that being healthy is a full-time job. Most people enjoy good health until about their high school years and then see it quickly unravel shortly thereafter. It's getting worse by the day in our country. I'm not saying you can never partake in yummy junk food once in a while, but let's be real for a minute. If you want to live a healthy life that does not require constant drug abuse and trips to the doctor, you are going to have to work at it. That's just the way it goes.

The payoff is incredible though. I love the fact that I can compete with kids half my age in just about any physical competition and destroy them! I am proud of the fact that I have taken care of myself and haven't treated my body like a human garbage dump. As I look to the future, I foresee myself being one of these people in their 70s and 80s out there running a 5K or 10K and still going strong. That's going to be me. I have vowed to myself and to God that I will do everything in my power to make that happen, and now I'm telling you.

You don't need to share my ambitions. You don't need to participate in martial arts, run in 5Ks, or be into bodybuilding, but do something. Find what motivates you. Find what you enjoy doing and do it. Make a commitment to yourself that you will stick with it for the rest of your life. You can have awesome health, you can have a beautiful body, and you can return to health! You can have it all.

Acknowledgments

I would like to thank all the people in my life who in some way either inspired or supported me in the writing of this book. It has been my experience in life that support and inspiration can come from either direct or indirect means. I am deeply grateful for all the experiences in my life that have led me to the writing of this book.

A very special thanks to:

My wife, Wendy, first and foremost. Your love, support, and inspiration are beyond what words can describe. I feel blessed to be walking this path with you. I am so grateful for you, my love. You are an incredible woman and I love you.

My boys, Alex, Nick, and Nolan. I draw inspiration from you in so many ways. I love you guys.

Mom and Dad, I love you and miss you.

My brother, Chris Kuhn. I love you.

The best in-laws and funniest people a man could ask for, Rose and Bill Ahler. I love you.

Rebecca Young and Ashley Digby. Your support and loyalty are priceless. I couldn't ask for a better team, and I am appreciative of you both every day of my life.

Tim Feuling. Thanks so much for writing a heartfelt foreword to this book and being a supportive mentor and friend.

Monica Sigmon. Thanks so much for the great photograph on my book cover.

Thank you to all the following people who have played important roles in my life, through personal mentoring, support, or leadership:

Dan Roose, Anthony Robbins, Dr. Dean Depice, Dr. Wayne Dyer, Dr. Deepak Chopra, Dr. Andy Barlow, Dr. Mike Johnson, Mary Jo Tate, Dr. David Simon, Daniel & Juliana Morris, Dr. Marcy Dionisio, Lisa Dionisio, Sue Wagner, Dr. Ben Lerner, Dr. Greg Loman, Dr. Mariella Loman, Dr. Dan Yachter, Dr. John Demartini, Mark Victor Hansen, and Napoleon Hill.

Last but not least, thank you, God, for showing me my vision and purpose in life and for giving me the inspiration and perseverance to see things through.

Return to
Health Seminars

Dr. Kuhn is now conducting Return to Health weekend seminars in various locations throughout the country. Visit our website to look for Return to Health seminars in your area.

Our seminars will be fully interactive seminars where you will learn firsthand how to apply the principles taught in this book. The topics covered will be totally congruent with what Dr. Kuhn has written about here.

Dr. Kuhn is a top level speaker and teacher in the healthcare industry and will lead you through day-to-day techniques of healthy living. You will be inspired to lead a better life and may gain a more thorough understanding of the Return to Health concepts presented here. Come and learn the most up to date information in healthcare, detox methods, visualization, healthy eating, proper exercise routines, stress management techniques, better sleeping habits, and using the law of attraction for success and health.

We hope to see you at a seminar soon!

Functional Medicine

Dr. Kuhn takes care of patients from all over the country in his home office. He will do a thorough health history, detailed neurological evaluation and complete metabolic assessment to get to the root cause of your health challenges.

Upon returning home, he will do his best to set you up with a functional medicine practitioner in your area after you have had your initial testing and recommendations. Visit our website to see if functional medicine can help you.

Dr. Kuhn will make the appropriate referral for medical evaluation if necessary.

About the Author

Dr. Robert Kuhn has been in full time practice since 1999. His wellness-based practice focuses on taking care of people with chronic conditions, autoimmunity, weight problems and numerous undiagnosed pain syndromes and health problems. Dr. Kuhn is Board Certified in Integrative Medicine and holds a diplomate in Whole Medical Systems. He has been helping patients regain their health utilizing functional medicine and functional neurology techniques in his practice for the past several years.

In 2008, Dr. Kuhn and his entire family experienced their own healthcare nightmare. After three years of misdiagnosis, functional medicine came to the rescue. This event caused Dr. Kuhn to shift the focus of his practice toward taking care of chronically ill people.

Dr. Kuhn lives with his wife and three children in Williamsburg, Virginia, where he maintains a very busy practice. He enjoys the study of personal development, traveling, public speaking and physical fitness. His personal mission is to help as many people as possible that suffer from chronic pain and chronic health problems and for he himself to be a prime example of optimal health.

Made in the USA
Middletown, DE
24 September 2019